Speech Therapy

A PRACTICAL APPROACH

Mark Hudson

Stanley Thornes (Publishers) Ltd

Text © Mark Hudson, 1998
Original line illustrations © Stanley Thornes (Publishers) Ltd, 1998

First published in 1998 by:
Stanley Thornes (Publishers) Ltd
Ellenborough House
Wellington Street
CHELTENHAM
GL50 1YW
United Kingdom

98 99 00 01 02 / 10 9 8 7 6 5 4 3 2 1

A catalogue record for this book is available from the British Library.

ISBN 0 7487 3374 4

Typeset by Northern Phototypesetting Co. Ltd, Bolton, Lancs.
Printed and bound in Great Britain
by Scotprint, Musselburgh

Contents

1 What is sports therapy?

After working through this chapter you will be able to:
➤ understand the role of sports therapy
➤ differentiate between sports therapy and traditional physiotherapy
➤ identify courses suitable to your requirements.

Sports therapy, in name at least, is a relatively new concept. In practice people have been attending to injured athletes, on the field and in treatment rooms, for as long as anyone can remember. We have all seen 'Mr Bucket and Sponge' running onto a football pitch and apparently 'healing' an injured player. These days we tend to be a little more scientific in our application.

What is a sports therapist?

A sports therapist might be someone capable of offering advice on safe exercise – or someone who delivers massage before and after a sporting event – or a highly trained practitioner able to recognise common orthopaedic conditions and soft tissue injuries as well as being able to complete a progressive and effective programme of treatment and rehabilitation.

Where do I start?

Identify what you want. Which appeals to you most?

- Expert in exercise
- Masseur
- Treater of injuries

You will need to be clear of your aims to find the right course of study. Choose carefully.

Some courses, called 'sports therapy' by some training companies, are no more than sports massage courses. The same principle applies to qualifications – one school's certificate is another's diploma because there is of yet no independent body to rule where one ends and the other begins.

Sports therapy currently operates on three levels:

1 The highest level are the courses taught by chartered physiotherapists. These have been developed from a clinical foundation.

2 Next are college courses. Their clinical content varies; they usually sit within the beauty therapy or massage department and have a massage and exercise background.

3 Finally there are people trained in massage who choose to be called sports therapists rather than massage therapists.

All three have their merits – you just need to choose the course that's right for you. Remember, you can always start with massage and build on that qualification later.

What should I be studying?

All clinically based sports therapy courses should include study in the following areas:

- extensive anatomy and physiology
- cause and prevention of injury
- pathology of injury
- patient/client assessment
- treatment planning and rehabilitation
- mechanical and electrical therapy
- cryotherapy
- bandaging and strapping
- codes of ethics and standards
- business management
- case studies and practical experience.

Sports massage is a much simpler course and focuses on manual massage techniques, together with appropriate anatomy and physiology. Sports massage is an excellent starting point for sports therapy.

Sports therapy – what is isn't

Sports therapy is *not* physiotherapy. As a sports therapist you are not qualified to treat medical conditions beyond the scope of those studied in your training. Physiotherapists currently study full time for three years before working in clinical practice – most often in the National Health Service.

Starting

Being a sports therapist is very rewarding, but there are no true short cuts to becoming one. As a sports therapist you are going to encounter many new words and ideas, and at times you'll look at this book and think it's been written in a foreign language. Be patient. If you don't understand something, go back and read it again. Don't panic if at first you don't understand – you will in time, although it won't happen overnight; it takes time to understand this new language. Whenever you encounter a new or unfamiliar word, look at the glossary or a medical dictionary. You might find it helpful to write the definition down or even to make up your own working glossary as you progress through the book.

Here is a brief glossary of terms to start you off. There is a more detailed glossary at the end of the book.

2

Glossary of terms

Term	Common meaning
Abduction	Movement of a part away from the body
Adduction	Movement of a part towards the body
Anterior	Situated towards the front
Articulation	The process of being united by a joint or joints
Atrophy	Reduction in size of a muscle or region of the body
Bursa	A small sac filled with synovial fluid that allows muscle or tendon to slide over bone
Crepitus	A grating sound or feeling sometimes found in fractures, tendonitis and joint pathologies
Dislocation	Displacement of one or more bones of a joint totally out of the natural position
Distal	Furthest from the centre (or midline) of the body
Dorsiflexion	Bending the foot towards its upper surface
Ecchymosis	Bleeding visible beneath skin, causing a blue or purple discoloration
Eversion	A turning outwards
Extension	Straightening out of a flexed joint
External rotation	Rotation of a body part away from the midline
Fascia	The fibrous tissue lying between muscles, forming the sheaths around muscles and other structures such as nerves and blood vessels
Flexion	Bending of a joint
Haemarthrosis	Blood within a joint
Haematoma	A collection of blood (usually clotted), which forms a mass within the tissues following trauma to the blood vessels
Haemorrhage	Escape of blood through damaged blood vessel walls
Hypertrophy	An increase in size of a body part
Hypothermia	Reduction of body temperature to below normal, which slows physiological processes
Inflammation	The reaction of tissues to injury. Characterised by heat, swelling, redness and pain
Internal rotation	Rotation of a body part towards the midline
Inversion	A turning inwards
Lateral	Away from the midline of the body
Ligament	A band of flexible tough fibrous tissue which connects bone to bone of joints
Manipulation	Skilled use of hands to move joints and muscles
Medial	Towards the midline of the body

Microtrauma	Minor, insignificant, injury. If it occurs repeatedly, microtrauma will give rise to an obvious injury
Neuromuscular	Pertaining to both nerves and muscles
Oedema	Excessive accumulation of fluid in tissues and joints
Plantar flexion	Bending the foot downwards towards the sole
Pronation	Turning of the palm of the hand downwards; lowering of the arch of the foot
Proprioception	Part of the nervous system which provides the appreciation of balance, equilibrium and changes in muscle length and joint position
Rehabilitation	Restoration of function to damaged areas of the body
Sprain	An injury to a ligament
Strain	An injury involving the muscle, tendon or musculotendinous unit
Subluxation	Incomplete or partial dislocation of a joint
Supination	The turning of the palm of the hand upwards; raising of the arch of the foot
Synovium	A membrane lining the joint capsule, bursa and tendon sheaths. The synovium produces the synovial fluid found in these structures
Tendon	A band of fibrous tissue attaching muscle to bone
Trauma	Injury to tissue caused by a mechanical or physical agent
Vascular	Pertaining to the blood vessels

2 Anatomy and physiology

After working through this chapter you will be able to:
- ➤ describe the main features of the musculoskeletal system
- ➤ describe the functions of the musculoskeletal system
- ➤ identify the differences between muscles, ligaments and tendons
- ➤ demonstrate and describe the role of each type of joint
- ➤ demonstrate the anatomical position of the body.

Traditionally, when studying anatomy and physiology you are required to study the major systems of the human body:

- the integumentary system
- the skeletal system
- the muscular system
- the nervous system
- the endocrine system
- the cardiovascular system
- the lymphatic and immune systems
- the respiratory system
- the digestive system
- the urinary system
- the reproductive system.

To study these in any depth is beyond the scope of this book. We will, however, be studying in some detail the **musculoskeletal system** – an appropriate combination of the skeletal and the muscular systems, including the ligaments and tendons.

The skeletal system

The human skeleton is composed of 206 bones, which are shaped according to their function. Bones may be:

- long, as in the arms and legs
- short, as in the ankles and wrists
- flat, as in the sternum and scapulae
- irregular, as in the vertebrae
- round, as in the patellae.

The bones of the arms, legs, shoulders, and pelvis make up the **appendicular skeleton**; the bones of the skull and face and the auditory ossicles, vertebrae, ribs, sternum and hyoid bone make up the **axial skeleton** (Figure 2.1)

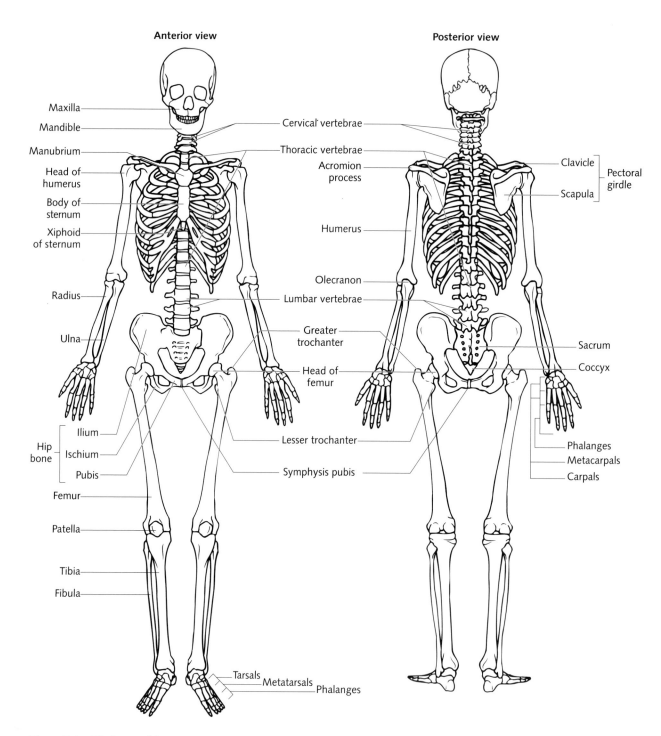

Figure 2.1 *The human skeleton*

Functions of bone

The five principal functions of bones are to:

- support the body, enabling you to stand erect
- protect the internal organs and tissues
- assist movement by co-ordination with muscles and joints
- provide storage areas (or reservoirs) for minerals
- serve as sites for formation of blood cells in the bone marrow (**haematopoiesis**).

haematopoiesis
production of blood cells;
occurs in red bone marrow

Skeletal growth

The skeleton develops in the growing fetus through a process called **osteogenesis**. The skeleton is completely formed by the end of the third month of gestation. After birth secondary centres develop in the **epiphyseal** regions, and bone growth proceeds from the end towards the centre of the bone. When the bone has reached its full size and growth ceases the epiphyseal growth centres are replaced by bone cells.

epiphyseal
responsible for the
lengthways growth of long
bones

While the bones are growing, they lengthen and the outer diameter increases slightly. New bone is continuously being deposited on the outer surfaces while the inner surfaces are reabsorbed, until the bone achieves its final shape. These formation – resorption processes help to remodel or shape the bone to maximise its load-bearing ability while minimising its weight.

Longitudinal bone growth and ossification usually continue in girls until about 15 years of age and in boys until age 16. However, bones continue to mature and develop their final shape until a person is 21 years of age – in both sexes with such regularity that a person's age can be fairly closely determined by X-ray examination.

Structure of bone tissue

Figure 2.2 shows the gross structure and individual parts of a long bone. The cartilage covering the epiphysis cushions the ends of the bone and provides protection during weight bearing and movement (Figure 2.3). The shaft is separated from the epiphysis by the growth plate and by nutrient arteries of the metaphysis. The shaft of the bone is composed of hard, dense bone cells called **compact bone**, whereas the ends of the bones are made up of soft, spongy bone cells called **cancellous bone**. Cancellous bone cells in the crest of the iliac bones, in the tibia, sternum and ends of the long bones contain red bone marrow for haematopoiesis. The shafts of the long bones contain yellow marrow cells, whose function is to replenish red marrow cells when necessary.

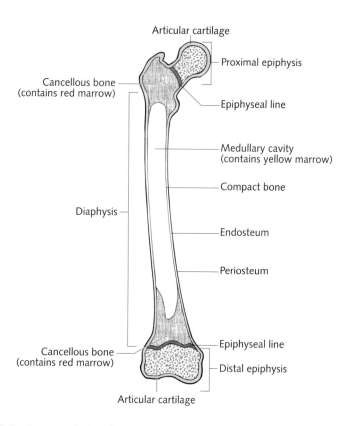

Articular cartilage

Proximal epiphysis

Cancellous bone
(contains red marrow)

Epiphyseal line

Medullary cavity
(contains yellow marrow)

Compact bone

Endosteum

Diaphysis

Periosteum

Cancellous bone
(contains red marrow)

Epiphyseal line

Distal epiphysis

Articular cartilage

Figure 2.2   *Structure of a long bone*

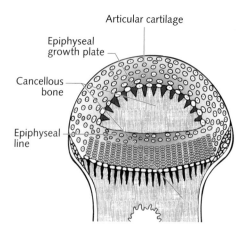

Articular cartilage

Epiphyseal
growth plate

Cancellous
bone

Epiphyseal
line

Figure 2.3   *Close-up of the epiphyseal region of bone*

Bone surfaces

Many of the surface features of bones can be seen in Figure 2.4. The surface of a bone has many prominences, which serve both as attachments for ligaments and tendons and to protect nerves and blood vessels.

Prominences may be:

- rounded, knuckle like protuberances (condyles)
- small, round projections (tubercles)
- large, irregular processes (trochanters)
- narrow ridges or crests (as seen in, for example, frontal bone and the iliac crest).

Projections may be transverse (transverse processes of vertebrae and ears), or they may extend posteriorly (posterior spinous processes) or anteriorly, as in the nasal cartilage.

Bones also contain:

- alveoli (sockets)
- fossae (depressions)
- fissures (narrow slits)
- foramina (openings for nerves, muscles and blood vessels)
- sinuses (cavities)
- sulci (grooves).

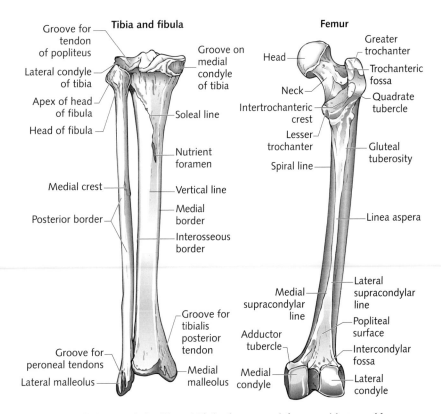

Figure 2.4 *The femur and the tibia and fibula show many of the external features of bone described in the text*

periosteum
the membrane that covers bone

The tough outer covering of bones (the **periosteum**) contains nutrient arteries to nourish the bone cells. Fibres in the periosteum, called Sharpey's fibres, penetrate the bone and hold the periosteum to the bone. The periosteal blood vessels communicate with vessels in the central canal of the Haversian system, which is the microscopic structural unit of compact bone.

ACTIVITY

Work with a partner to find the following: clavicle, sternum, head of humerus, olecranon, iliac crest, greater trochanter, medial epicondyle of femur, lateral epicondyle of femur, head of fibula, patella, medial malleolus, lateral malleolus and calcaneus.

The Haversian system

The Haversian system is composed of four parts:

1 lamellae – connective layers of cylindrical, calcified matrix cells aligned parallel to the shaft of the bone

2 lacunae – small cavities or spaces in lamellae that are filled with tissue fluids and bone cells (osteocytes)

3 canaliculi – very small canals that connect with larger canals called Haversian canals

4 Haversian canals – channels extending lengthways through the centre of each Haversian system; they contain blood vessels to provide nutrients and to remove wastes produced by bone growth and resorption.

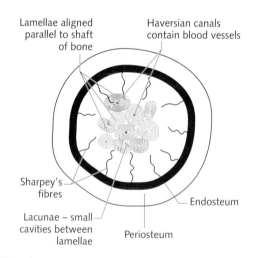

Lamellae aligned parallel to shaft of bone

Haversian canals contain blood vessels

Sharpey's fibres

Endosteum

Lacunae – small cavities between lamellae

Periosteum

Figure 2.5 *The Haversian system*

Bone formation and resorption

Bones are living structures and are continuously being formed and resorbed. Bone formation and resorption are caused by the actions of

osteoblasts and **osteoclasts**. The main cells forming the bone, the **osteocytes**, develop from mature osteoblasts, spindle-shaped cells found in the **endosteum** and beneath the periosteum of bones. The main function of the osteocytes is to maintain the bone structure.

Bone is constantly being formed and resorbed, in conjunction with other processes involving calcium metabolism, to prevent the bones from becoming excessively thick or thin. Approximately 98% of the body's extracellular calcium is contained in the bones. Concentrations of calcium and phosphate in the body are kept relatively stable by regulation by parathyroid hormone (from the parathyroid glands), which affects their absorption in the intestines, and their retention or excretion through the kidneys.

When the level of calcium in the serum is low the parathyroid glands produce parathyroid hormone, which stimulates the osteoclasts to break down bone, releasing calcium phosphate crystals into the blood and increasing serum calcium concentrations. In addition to this, the intestinal ion transport system absorbs more calcium from food, moving the calcium ions from the gut to the blood. The renal tubules are also stimulated to retain instead of excrete calcium – further raising serum calcium levels (but concurrently reducing the retention or resorption of phosphate). Through these processes, the levels of calcium in the serum remain relatively constant, and bones remain strong with relatively stable calcium content.

Vitamin D is involved in the absorption of calcium and phosphorus from the intestine. A deficiency of either vitamin D or sunshine (which is needed to activate conversion of sterol precursors to vitamin D in the skin) can cause loss of calcium from the bones – a condition known in children as rickets and in adults as osteomalacia.

Haematopoiesis

Haematopoiesis (sometimes known as haemopoiesis) is the process of producing and developing blood cells. It takes place in the marrow of the bones. As mentioned earlier, there are two types of bone marrow: red and yellow.

In the red marrow in the cancellous areas of the bones (particularly in the sternum, iliac crests and tibias), red blood cells, white blood cells and megakaryocytes, the 'mother cells' of platelets develop from primitive **'stem' cells**.

Hematopoiesis requires haemopoietin, which is produced in the kidneys, as a catalyst to stimulate cell production.

The only function for the yellow marrow is to transform into red marrow to assist with haematopoiesis at times of stress.

---

osteoblasts
cells responsible for synthesis, deposition and mineralisation of bone; mature osteoblasts can develop into osteocytes

osteoclasts
cells responsible for removal of bone tissue

osteocytes
the main cells forming the structure of bone, responsible for maintaining bone structure

endosteum
the membrane that lines the marrow cavity of bones

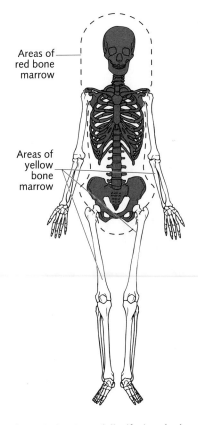

Areas of red bone marrow

Areas of yellow bone marrow

Figure 2.6 *General distribution of red and yellow bone marrow*

The muscular system

Muscles are masses of tissues that cover bones. They have the following functions:

- to provide bulk to the body
- to help hold the body parts together
- to help move one or more parts from place to place.

Muscles interact with nerves, minerals, skin, and other connective tissues to bring about muscle contraction for movement in space.

There are three types of muscles:

- skeletal
- smooth
- cardiac

Although it is important for the therapist to have a thorough understanding of all muscle types, in this book we will concern ourselves only with skeletal muscle.

Skeletal muscles

Skeletal muscle (see Figures 2.7–2.9) makes up 40–45% of the body's

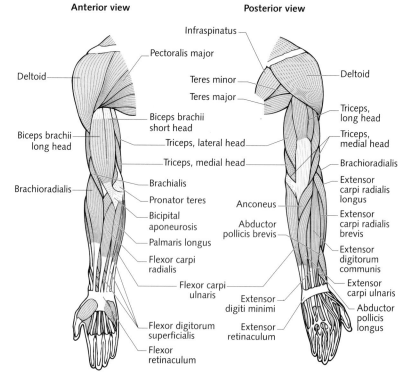

Figure 2.7 *Muscles of the arm*

12

weight. It contains muscle tissue, nerves, blood vessels and connective tissue elements. Skeletal muscles vary in size from very small (e.g. teres minor) to the large muscle masses, such as the thigh muscles. Skeletal muscle may be short, blunt, long and narrow, triangular, quadrilateral, flat, bulky or irregular in shape.

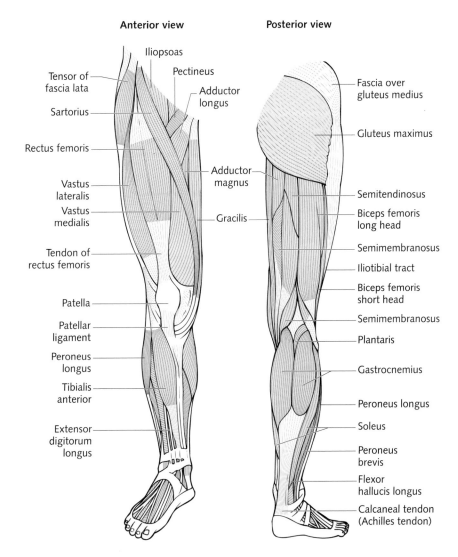

Anterior view

Tensor of fascia lata
Sartorius
Rectus femoris
Vastus lateralis
Vastus medialis
Tendon of rectus femoris
Patella
Patellar ligament
Peroneus longus
Tibialis anterior
Extensor digitorum longus

Iliopsoas
Pectineus
Adductor longus
Adductor magnus
Gracilis

Posterior view

Fascia over gluteus medius
Gluteus maximus
Semitendinosus
Biceps femoris long head
Semimembranosus
Iliotibial tract
Biceps femoris short head
Semimembranosus
Plantaris
Gastrocnemius
Peroneus longus
Soleus
Peroneus brevis
Flexor hallucis longus
Calcaneal tendon (Achilles tendon)

***Figure* 2.8**   *Muscles of the leg*

oblique
slanting or indirect

Skeletal muscle fibres may be arranged parallel to the long axis of the bone to which they are attached, or **obliquely** attached. They may be curved (as seen in sphincters), pennate (like feathers in a plume), or bipennate (double-feathered). The arrangements of the fibres in specific muscles helps to produce that particular muscle's optimum contraction.

> **fascia**
> *outer connective tissue*

Muscles are attached at each end to a bone, ligament, tendon or **fascia**. One end of the muscle, the more fixed end, is called the **origin**; the more moveable end is the muscle **insertion**.

Skeletal muscles may be red or white:

- Red muscles get their colour from the pigment myoglobin. Closely related to haemoglobin, myoglobin acts as a temporary oxygen store for the muscle. Red muscle fibres carry out slower, more sustained movements than white muscle.
- White muscle fibres contain less myoglobin. They react rapidly when stimulated.

Normally, muscles are full-bellied and supple, but as they age they lose some fibres through degeneration. The lost fibres may be replaced with fibrous connective tissue. Loss of muscle fibre and an increase in connective tissue cause loss of full muscle strength, which is noticeable in older people.

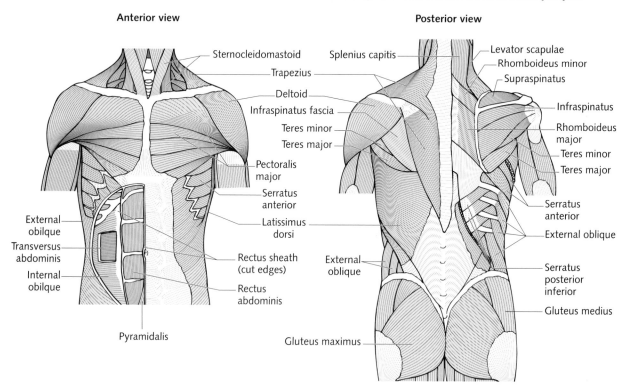

Figure 2.9 *Muscles of the trunk and pelvis*

Muscle fibres

All muscles are composed of the basic cellular unit, called the muscle fibre, which is a cell containing many structures (Figure 2.10).

> **fasciculus**
> *a small bundle or cluster, especially of nerve or muscle fibres*

Skeletal muscles are composed of many fibres. Some muscle fibres are elongated cells that may extend the entire length of a particular muscle. Muscle fibres are arranged in bundles, called **fasciculi**, and each fasciculus is surrounded by connective tissue – the **endomysium**. The endomysium connects with connective tissue partitions called **perimysia**, which in turn are connected to the outer muscle covering (the **epimysium**). These three connective tissues provide pathways for nerves and blood vessels.

striated
arranged in parallel lines

sarcomere
a contractile unit of striated muscle fibre

Skeletal muscles are described as **striated**, because alternating light and dark bands, or striations, can be seen in muscle tissue under a light microscope (Figure 2.10). The light bands are known as the I bands and the dark ones as the A bands (Figure 2.12). Under an electron microscope, each I band can be seen to be crossed by a dark area (known as the Z line) and each A band has a lighter area within it, called the H band. Each H band has a dark streak, called the M line. The area of muscle fibre between two Z lines is called a **sarcomere**. As was shown in Figure 2.10, the sarcomeres contain two types of protein fibre – actin and myosin. These filaments run close to each other but are not attached because another protein, called tropomyosin, is bound to the myosin and prevents it forming bonds with actin. The H band contains only myosin and the A band contains both actin and myosin.

sarcolemma
the cell membrane of a muscle fibre

sarcoplasm
the cytoplasm of a muscle fibre

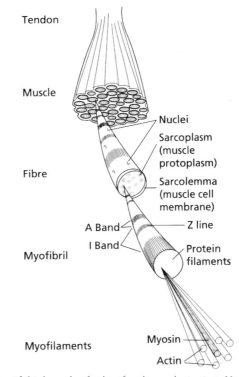

Figure 2.10 *Skeletal muscle, showing the microscopic structure. Note the striations in the fibre and the myofibril. These are alternating light and dark bands caused by the geometric arrangement of the filaments in actin and myosin.*

endomysium
invagination of the perimysium that separates each individual muscle fibre

perimysium
invagination of the epimysium that divides muscles into bundles

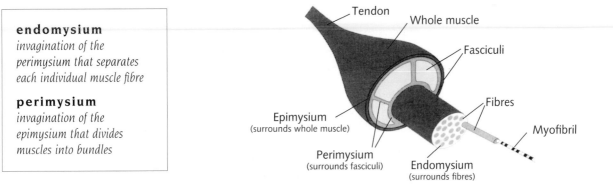

Figure 2.11 *Anatomy of skeletal muscle*

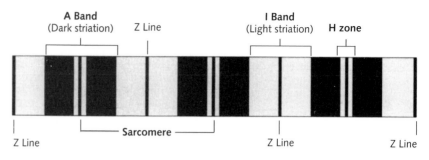

Figure 2.12 *Striations in a muscle fibre*

Muscle contraction and relaxation

Contraction of the muscle takes place in the sarcomere. An electrical impulse passes along a motor nerve to the motor endplate (where the nerve meets the muscle). This causes release of a neurotransmitter (acetylcholine) at the junction, which passes across from the nerve to the muscle and stimulates release of calcium in the sarcoplasm.

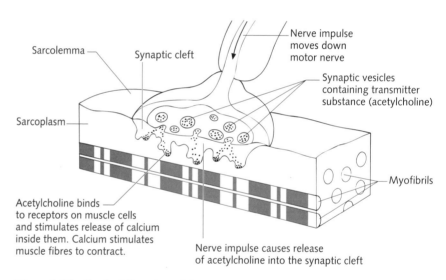

Figure 2.13 *Events at the motor endplate*

The calcium binds with troponin, another protein, which is normally bound to actin when muscles are at rest. Formation of calcium–troponin molecules changes the tropomyosin on the myosin fibres so that they are now able to bind with the actin fibres. When these two fibres interact the thin fibres of actin are pulled towards the centre of each sarcomere, shortening the muscle fibre – this is muscle contraction.

When a muscle contracts the following can be observed under the microscope:

- The width of the I band decreases (this area of the sarcomere contains only actin filaments).
- The width of the A band does not alter (this area of the sarcomere is equal to the length of the myosin filaments).

16

- The H band disappears (this area of the sarcomere contains only myosin filaments).

The explanation of what is happening in the sarcomere during muscle contraction can be seen in Figure 2.14.

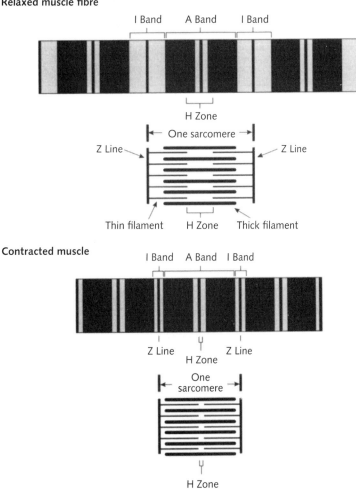

Figure 2.14 *Changes at the sarcomere during muscle contraction*

The muscle must be able to relax as well as contract. Muscle relaxation is currently thought to be brought about by separation of the calcium-troponin combination. When this occurs, the calcium ions re-enter the muscle sarcoplasm and the tropomyosin reforms its usual bonds with the myosin filaments so that they can no longer interact with the actin filaments. This is thought to be the normal state in relaxed muscles between stimuli.

Muscular energy

Most of the energy for muscle contraction comes from hydrolysis of the high-energy bonds in **ATP**:

ATP

adenosine triphosphate, a form of chemical energy found in all cells. When ATP is broken down to adenosine diphosphate (ADP) and phosphate energy is released

ATP → ADP + phosphate + energy.

Other energy sources are phosphocreatine, a protein found only in muscle tissues, and oxygen, which aids contraction by oxidising the lactic acid that results from anaerobic hydrolysis of the high-energy ATP bonds.

Muscle spasm versus muscle twitch

A *muscle spasm* results from involuntary contraction of a muscle or group of muscles. It is caused by repetitive activation of entire motor units, which in turn is caused by the repetitive firing of a motor nerve.

A *muscle twitch* occurs when a stimulus is attained. All muscle fibres associated with the stimulated nerve contract and then relax.

An isotonic (or concentric) twitch causes the muscle to change length when constant tension is applied throughout its contraction. This is the most common type of muscle contraction. An isometric twitch is a contraction in which the muscle does not alter in length, even with a sudden increase in muscle tension. This types of contraction occurs when a muscle is working against a resistance it can't overcome.

Muscle tone

Tone helps muscles to passively elongate or stretch and ensures rapid reaction to an external stimulus. It results from a continuous flow of stimuli from the spinal cord to each motor unit. Muscle tone can be increased or decreased, depending on the activity within the nervous system. Tone is increased in anxiety states and decreased during restful periods.

ACTIVITY

Work in pairs.

1 Using Figures 2.7–2.9, find the following muscles on your partner: deltoid, biceps brachii, brachioradialis, triceps, pectoralis major, pectoralis minor, sternocleidomastoid, serratus anterior, external oblique, rectus abdominis, levator scapulae, teres major, teres minor, latissimus dorsi, rhomboids, gluteus maximus, gluteus medius, sartorius, rectus femoris, vastus lateralis, vastus medialis, tibialis anterior, semitendinosus, biceps femoris, semimembranosus, iliotibial tract, gastrocnemius and soleus.
2 Try finding:
   - the muscle belly
   - the origin
   - the insertion
3 Get your partner to move the associated limb and make a note of the movement available in each muscle. This is an activity that you should practice often and on as many different people as possible.

Ligaments

Ligaments are tough, relatively long bands of dense connective tissues that hold bones to bones. They are composed of type I collagen fibres (see page 22) arranged in parallel bundles, which gives them great strength but limited ability to extend. Ligaments may:

- encircle a joint to add strength and stability – as they do around the hip joint
- hold obliquely or parallel to the ends of bones across the joint – as they do in and around the knee joint (Figure 2.15).

Ligaments provide the greatest stability to the joint when they are taut (under strain). They allow movement in some directions while restricting movements in other directions. Ligaments may be injured by partial tears, called **sprains**, or they may be torn loose from their attachment to the bones. Such an injury is called an **avulsion**.

sprain
forcible wrenching or twisting of a joint, causing partial rupture or other injury to its attachments without dislocation

avulsion
pulling away

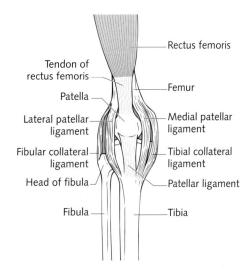

Rectus femoris

Tendon of rectus femoris

Femur

Patella

Lateral patellar ligament

Medial patellar ligament

Fibular collateral ligament

Tibial collateral ligament

Head of fibula

Patellar ligament

Fibula

Tibia

Figure 2.15 *Ligaments and tendons of the knee joint*

Tendons

Tendons are very strong, tough, long strands or cords of dense connective tissues that form at the ends of muscles (see Figure 2.15). The fibres of tendons are arranged in longitudinal and parallel rows into non-elastic cords which have high tensile strength. Tendons can transmit great forces from contractile muscles to bone or cartilage while remaining undamaged themselves. Tendons are composed of type I collagen fibres, which give them their strength. The Achilles tendon is the longest and largest tendon in the body, being 10–14 cm long. Other tendons may be only 2–3 cm in length.

ACTIVITY	Using your partner, find the Achilles tendon, note its origin and its point of insertion into the calcaneum.

PROGRESS CHECK	1 What is the function of a ligament?
	2 What is the function of a tendon?

Cartilage

Cartilage is a semi-smooth layer of elastic, resilient supporting tissue at the ends of bones (see Figure 2.2). Cartilage forms a cap over the bone end, to protect and support to the bone during weight-bearing activity.

Functions of cartilage

Cartilage absorbs weight and shock due to weight-bearing exercise, thus avoiding stress and strain on a joint and helping to prevent injury to joints and bones.

Structure of cartilage

Adult cartilage is made up of cells called **chondrocytes**, which are usually arranged in clusters. Between the clusters of chondrocytes are 'ground substances' of complex protein–carbohydrate molecules. These give cartilage its elasticity.

perichondrium
the membrane that covers cartilage

The outer surfaces of cartilage are undulating, with small depressions and valleys. The area of cartilage nearest the bone end is the **perichondrium**; it contains blood vessels to bring nutrients to the cartilage and to remove waste materials.

The thickness of cartilage varies from 2 to 4 cm, depending on the area within a joint, and the particular joint. The colour of cartilage varies from shades of white to yellow.

synovial fluid
a fluid within the capsule of a joint that nourishes and lubricates the articular cartilage

The outer cartilage layers have no blood vessels of their own – they receive their nourishment from the **synovial fluid** that is forced into the elastic, spongy cartilage layers during weight bearing and other joint movements.

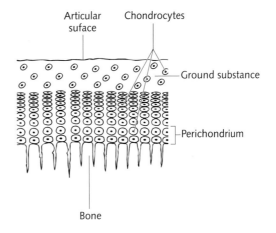

Figure 2.16 *The structure of adult cartilage*

Damage to cartilage

Joint movement and weight bearing are essential for cartilage to remain healthy. It will shrink and atrophy if the joint is not used, because the cells will not be replenished with nutrients from the synovial fluid. Weight-bearing exercise and joint movements keep cartilage from becoming thin, unhealthy, or damaged, conditions that could eventually lead to degenerative joint disease.

Cartilage can wear unevenly and may fray if the joints are not stable, anatomically correct (i.e. in the right places) or normally shaped.

When cartilage cells are moderately or severely damaged and die, they are replaced with new cells if the area is small. If the area of damage is large the dead cells may be replaced with fibrous tissue and become scars. Scarred cartilage is no longer spongy or resilient and is therefore less able to withstand loading, stress, or strain than healthy cartilage.

Types of cartilage

Hyaline cartilage

Hyaline cartilage (also called articular cartilage) is bluish white and translucent. The collagen fibres within it are arranged in an interlacing network. Water constitutes 70–80% of the net weight of adult hyaline cartilage, giving it great elasticity, sponginess and mouldability. Hyaline cartilage is found over the ends of bones of synovial joints, in the walls of the trachea, in the larynx and nasal septum, and over the ends of the ribs.

Fibrous cartilage

Fibrous cartilage (also known as fibrocartilage) is white and is made up of thick bundles of collagen fibres, which give it great strength. Fibrocartilage acts as a shock absorber. It is found in the symphysis pubis and between each vertebra, as well as in tendons and ligaments of synovial joints.

Yellow cartilage

Yellow (elastic) cartilage has a dense network of collagen fibres, giving it great flexibility and strength. It is easily bent but just as easily returns to its original shape. Yellow cartilage is found in the outer ear, epiglottis and the eustachian tubes.

PROGRESS CHECK

1 What is the function of cartilage?
2 Where would you expect to find cartilage?
3 Name two different types of cartilage.

Collagen

Collagen is the major supporting element in **connective tissues**, making up approximately half of the total body protein in adults. It is a fibrous protein, made up of three individual protein strands that are coiled tightly throughout the fibre. The structure is stabilised by hydrogen bonds between the protein chains. This coiling gives collagen its flexibility and resilience.

Many types of collagen are known, but there are three major types: type I, type II, or type III collagen.

Type I collagen

Type I collagen is found in all major **connective tissues** – tendons, bones, cornea of the eye, dentine of the teeth, and in the fibrocartilage between the vertebrae and in the symphysis pubis. Because type I collagen distends very little under mechanical stress, it gives strength to tendons and ligaments in and around joints.

Type II collagen

Type II is the major form of collagen found in hyaline cartilage. Its special properties add mouldability, flexibility and sponginess to the strength of the cartilage.

Type III collagen

Type III is the most distensible collagen. It is found in the walls of blood vessels, skin and the wall of the uterus – organs that need to distend to function normally.

> **connective tissue**
> *the most abundant of the four basic tissue types within the body – its principal function is to bind and support*

Joints

Joints are articulations – where bones are joined, or where two surfaces of bones come together. Joints help to hold the bones firmly together while permitting movement. Joints may be classified by the type of material between the bones or by the degree of movement available at the joint into:

- fibrous
- cartilaginous or
- synovial

joints, or:

- immovable (synarthrotic)
- slightly moveable (amphiarthrotic) or
- freely moveable (diarthrotic)

joints.

Types of joints

Type of joint	Description
Freely moveable (diarthrotic, or synovial) joints	
Uniaxial: permit movement in one axis and in only one plane	
Hinge	Permits back and forth extension and flexion. Examples are the knee, elbow and finger joints
Pivot	Permits movements of one bone articulating with a ring or notch of another bone. Examples: the projection of the second cervical vertebra articulates with a ring-shaped portion of the first cervical vertebra; the head of the radius articulates with the radial notch of the ulna
Biaxial: permit movement around two perpendicular axes in two perpendicular planes	
Saddle	Saddle-shaped bone ends articulate with each other. These joints are found only in the base of each thumb
Condyloid	The condyle of one bone fits into the elliptical portion of its articulating bone. Examples are seen in the distal end of the radius, which articulates with three wrist bones; the condyles of the occipital bone, which fit into elliptical depressions in the atlas
Multiaxial: permit movement in three or more planes and around three or more axes	
Ball and socket	Spheroid or ball-shaped bone fits into a concave curved area of its articulating bone. Examples: hip and shoulder joints
Gliding	Permits movement along various axes through relatively flat articulating surfaces. Examples: joints between two vertebrae
Slightly moveable (amphiarthrotic) joints	
Symphysis	Permits limited movement between the bones. Examples include the symphysis pubis, intervertebral joints and the manubriosternal joint
Immovable (synarthrotic) joints	
Suture	Fibrous tissue projections that interlock between articulating bones with only a thin layer of fibrous tissue separating them. The bones of the skull are held together by suture joints.
Syndesmosis	Ligaments connect two articulating bones – for example between the distal ends of the radius and ulna; between the distal ends of the tibia and fibula
Gomphoses	A fibrous membrane holds the root of a tooth in the alveolar process of the maxilla or mandible, forming a joint

PROGRESS CHECK   Give two examples of each of the following joints: ball and socket, hinge, gliding, pivot.

Most joints are diarthrotic joints. They are also known as *synovial* joints, because they are lined with a synovial membrane. The following features are found in a synovial joint:

- bones
- cartilage covering the ends of bones
- ligaments that hold the bones together
- synovial fluid
- blood vessels
- lymphatics
- nerves.

Some synovial joints, such as the knee, also have a disc, called a meniscus, which is a pad of cartilage that cushions the joint (see Figure 2.17). Synovial joints have a casing or covering surrounding them, called the joint capsule, which is an extension of the periosteum of the articulating bones. Ligaments also encase the capsule to add strength.

The amphiarthrotic joints are connected by cartilage, which permits slight

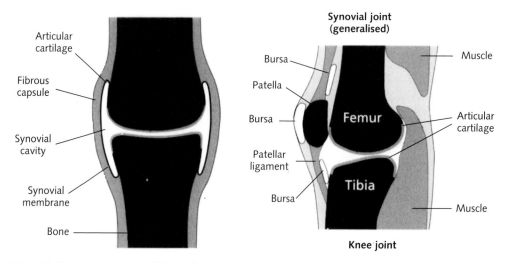

Figure 2.17   A *typical synovial joint – the knee*

movement between them. Examples of such joints are: the symphysis pubis, the manubriosternal joint (the attachments of the sternum to the first ten ribs), and the intervertebral joints.

Immovable joints are connected by *sutures* or fibrous tissues between the bones; this arrangement holds the bones so tightly together that no movement can occur between them.

Movement of joints

The degree of movement of a joint is called its *range of motion* (ROM). Only the synovial joints have more than one ROM (these are shown in Figure 2.18).

24

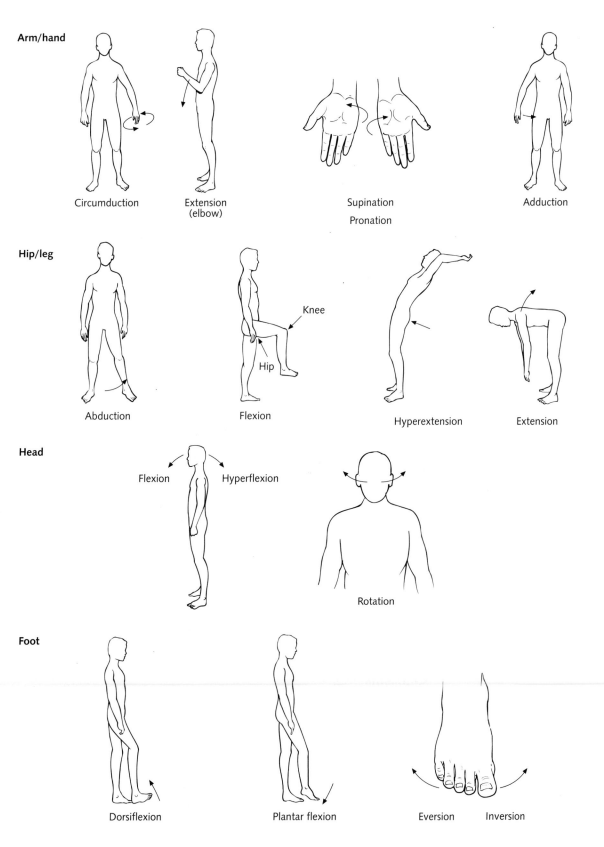

Figure 2.18   *Movements provided by synovial joints*

Types of movement

Type	Explanation
Angular: movements that change the angle between articulating bones	
Flexion	Bending forward, which decreases the angle between the bones
Extension	Bending backwards, which increases the angle between the bones
Abduction	Moving a part away from the midline of the body
Adduction	Moving a part towards the midline of the body
Plantar flexion	Stretching the foot and toes down and back, which increases the angle between the top of the foot and the front of the leg
Dorsiflexion	Flexing or tilting the foot and toes upwards towards the leg, which decreases the angle between the foot and the front of the leg
Hyperextension	Stretching an extended part beyond its normal position
Circular: movement around an axis	
Rotation	Moving or pivoting a bone on its own axis, as in side-to-side movement of the head
Circumduction	Moving a part so that its distal end forms a circular movement while the rest of the movement forms a cone, as in 'winding up' to throw a ball
Supination	Turning the palm upwards while rotating the forearm outwards
Pronation	Turning the palm downwards while rotating the forearm inwards
Gliding: movement of one joint surface over another without any circular or angular movement	
Special movements	
Elevation	Moving a part upwards, or lifting it
Depression	Moving a part downwards, or lowering it
Inversion	Turning the sole of the foot inwards
Eversion	Turning the sole of the foot outwards
Protraction	Moving a part forwards
Retraction	Moving a part backwards
Opposition	Moving parts together, as in bringing the thumb to touch a finger

ACTIVITY

Physically work your way through each movement, using the examples given to familiarise yourself with each.

Synovium

The synovium is the membrane that lines the inner surfaces of synovial joints (see Figure 2.17) and forms from cells within the inner layer of a joint capsule. It has numerous **villus** folds that contain blood vessels and lymphatic channels. The cells that form the synovial membrane are made up primarily of type I collagen. The blood vessels in the synovial folds are derived from type III collagen, which gives them distensibility.

The villus folds in the synovial membrane are filled with synovial fluid. This is secreted from the membrane to bathe and lubricate the joint and articular cartilage, aid joint movements, provide nutrients and oxygen to

villus
mucosal cells containing connective tissue, blood and lymphatic vessels

the joint tissues, and carry out phagocytic and other immunological functions within the joint.

Bursa

The bursae (see Figure 2.17) are sacs or cavities that are lined with synovial membrane and contain synovial fluid. They serve as cushioning areas between tendons and bones, tendons and ligaments or between other tissues where friction might occur. Bursae are musculoskeletal tissues, but pressure or friction can cause a new bursa to develop – as for example, the bursa that forms over a bunion in a hallux valgus deformity of the metatarsophalangeal joint.

KEY TERMS

You need to know what these words mean. Go back through the chapter or check the glossary to find out.

Abduction	Flexion	Pronation
Adduction	Insertion	Strain
Circumduction	Inversion	Symphysis
Dorsiflexion	Origin	Taut
Eversion	Plantar flexion	Tensile strength

---

3 Pathology of injury and repair – the healing process

After working through this chapter you will be able to:
- ➤ describe and understand the main features of the healing process
- ➤ describe and understand the role each part plays in the overall process
- ➤ explain the difference between healing by first intention and healing by second intention
- ➤ list factors that could affect the healing process
- ➤ understand the importance of scar control and appropriate patient management.

Most sports injuries are not generally serious – the damage to tissues is usually slight and the healing capacity good. In spite of this, the healing process often takes longer than we would like. The extra time needed to heal completely often conflicts with the patient's eagerness to return to sport at the highest level of performance possible as quickly as possible.

Because most sports injuries involve damage to soft tissue (ligaments, muscles, tendons, skin etc.), it is essential to understand the process of healing and repair. The fact is, wound healing is at best imperfect and the implications of this deficiency are vital for people playing sport. An appreciation and understanding of this point may be the key to the successful management of soft tissue sporting injuries.

The process of the formation of scar tissue, and its associated properties, is a particular aspect of wound healing not often satisfactorily understood.

The purpose of this chapter is to provide a rationale for the treatment of wound healing problems, based on the knowledge of the mechanisms involved in connective tissue repair and specific clinical observations.

The subject will be considered under four headings:
- inflammation and repair
- factors affecting wound healing
- healing of specific tissues
- scar tissue and patient management.

Inflammation and repair

The most common cause of injury in sport is trauma, either from external (extrinsic) force or from continual repetitive stress (intrinsic force). Other causes of injury are:

- chemical agents (stings, acids, etc.)
- extremes of heat and cold
- bacterial and viral infections
- all types of immunological reactions.

Wound healing is a sequence of events:

- inflammation
- fibroplasia (the growth of a fibrous tissue scar)
- remodelling.

Inflammation

Inflammation is best defined as the local reaction of **vascularised** tissue to injury. It is an essential check on bacterial infections; wounds and injuries would never heal without the inflammatory reaction, and it is an essential step in the process of repair.

On the other hand, inflammation is potentially harmful. With chronic inflammatory conditions or large wounds, reparative efforts often lead to disfiguring scars and **fibrous bonds** that limit the mobility and function of joints and organs.

The local clinical signs of inflammation are:

- heat
- redness
- swelling
- pain
- loss of function.

Immediately after injury **vasoconstriction occurs**. This is a minimal and inconsistent reaction, and is immediately followed by **vasodilation**, which increases the blood flow to the area and is the cause of the heat and redness.

The swelling is largely caused by fluid, plasma proteins and cells escaping from the blood vessel into the **perivascular tissues** as the blood vessels lose their normal ability to retain fluids and cells. White blood cells concentrate at the site.

The white blood cells are the major contributors to the body's defence mechanisms, so their concentration at the injury site helps to prevent invasion by infectious organisms.

Pain associated with injury is caused by a number of factors:

---

vascularised
containing blood

fibrous bond
a bond that allows little or no movement

REMEMBER

The inflammatory reaction is an essential step in the process of repair

---

vasoconstriction
decrease in size or tightening of blood vessels

vasodilation
increase in size or widening of blood vessels

perivascular tissue
tissue surrounding blood vessels

---

histamine
chemical released when cells are injured; results in vasodilation, increased permeability of blood vessels

ischaemia
lack of blood supply

- pressure on nerve endings due to the swelling
- release of certain body chemicals, particularly **histamines**, at the injury site
- **ischaemia** caused by damage to the local blood vessels.

PROGRESS CHECK

- Wound healing is a sequence of three events. What are they?
- What are the local signs of inflammation?

Fibroplasia

Fibroplasia (the process of wound repair) is a sequence of events which leads to the formation of a fibrous tissue scar. Soft tissue injuries can be repaired in two ways:

- primary (first) intention
- secondary (second) intention.

epithelial cells
cells that form the tissue of glands, the outer part of the skin and lining of blood vessels

Healing by first intention

A clean wound with even and closely opposed edges heals by first intention, or primary healing. The **epithelial** cells of the outer surface of the cut edge migrate and proliferate rapidly to bridge the gap, as shown in Figure 3.1.

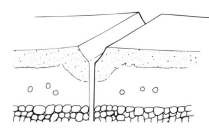

a   A clean wound caused by surgery or a cut

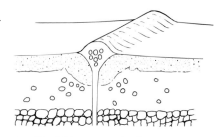

b   After 24 hours granulocytes, monocytes and lymphocytes accumulate to form an endothelium

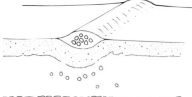

c   After 10–15 days, capillary growth is proceeding upwards from the subcutaneous tissue. Fibrosis (scarring) is far advanced. Scab falls off

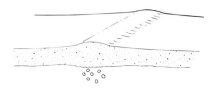

d   Months or years later a fine lamina of fibrous tissue marks the wound site

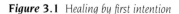

Figure 3.1 *Healing by first intention*

endothelium
tissue that lines the blood vessels and lymphatic vessels

Within 24 hours of the injury, large numbers of granulocytes, monocytes and lymphocytes (types of white blood cells) accumulate. By the end of the second day a smooth lining or **endothelium** has formed, By the third day small blood vessels (capillaries) sprout and by the fifth day an extensive network of **reticular fibres** has formed. Most of the collagen fibres are laid down during the second week after injury.

At first, the scar has many blood vessels and appears red, and on cold days, blue. After some months only a fine lamina of fibrous tissues marks the original site of the wound.

Healing by second intention

Healing by second intention occurs when there is a gaping wound with edges that cannot be approximated (Figure 3.2).

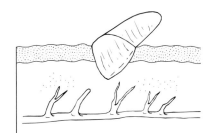

a Immediately (within 5 minutes), fibrinogen clots on the surface covering the wound. The wound cavity is filled with a blood clot

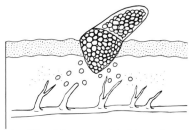

b After 6 days, granulated tissue forms at the base of the wound site

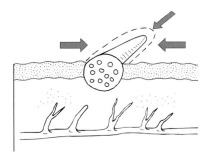

c Three weeks after injury, macrophages and fibroblasts from fibrous granulation tissue heal from the bottom and the sides upwards to create an elevation. As the wound closes, the surrounding tissue contracts

Figure 3.2 *Healing by second intention*

macrophages
cells that engulf and digest foreign bodies in the blood, such as bacteria and cell debris

fibroblasts
cells that synthesise the extracellular matrix of connective tissue

Immediately after injury, a sequence of reactions occurs in the blood that results in conversion of the soluble blood protein fibrinogen into insoluble fibrin. The fibrin rapidly forms a transparent clot, covering and sealing the wound. By five to six days, the surface appears red and finely granular. Each of the granules consists of a core of new capillaries, the growth of which raises the enveloping mantle of **macrophages**, **fibroblasts** and other cells into a small elevation, or scab.

| PROGRESS CHECK | How do healing by first intention and healing by second intention differ? |

Remodelling

The third stage of repair is the remodelling phase. This phase is characterised by:

- reduction in size of the wound surface
- increase in the strength of the scar
- alteration of the fibre structure.

Contraction of the wound starts as soon as the regeneration of the granulation tissue has occurred, and continues for as long as the elasticity of the surrounding fibres allows. Wound contraction is a function of specialised contractile fibroblasts, a variety of the cells which synthesise collagen fibres.

In the early stages of healing, the strength of a wound relates directly to the quality of the collagen present. After two or three weeks of healing, further gains in strength are determined by qualitative changes in these fibres. The strength gain at this later stage is thought to be due to two factors:

- intramolecular and intermolecular cross-linking of the collagen fibres
- remodelling caused by dissolution and reforming of the collagen fibres, to give a stronger, more efficient weave.

| PROGRESS CHECK | What are the three characteristics of the remodelling phase? |

Old fibres of collagen are continuously being broken down and new ones formed, although the quality remains constant. The rate of this turnover in the first three months is related to the increase in strength of the scar.

The remodelling phase has the most important implications for the management of soft-tissue injuries – the rigidity, loss of extensibility and lack of tensile strength of the scar tissue. These factors are discussed in depth later in this chapter (see page 37)

Factors affecting wound healing

The final nature and quality of the wound healing product depends on a number of factors, including:

- blood supply to the area
- age of the patient
- administration of steroids
- activity
- size of the wound
- swelling.

Blood supply

Research has shown that the rate and quality of wound repair is directly proportional to the oxygen supply to the tissues. As tissues are supplied with oxygen by the blood, an adequate blood supply must be present to allow healing to proceed normally. Poor circulation may slow healing down. Unfortunately, the original injury often damages local circulation, so optimal conditions for tissue nutrition are achieved only if:

- blood supply to the area is adequate
- vasoconstriction is minimised
- overall blood volume is maintained
- fluid overload and tissue oedema are avoided.

---

metabolic rate
the speed at which reactions occur in a cell

Heating the tissues has been found to increase blood supply and aid the healing process. One degree of heating increases the **metabolic rate** of a cell by about 13%, allowing faster exchange of nutrients and waste materials. Heat from an infrared lamp, hot water bottle, warm bath or shower can be applied at home, in the treatment room or the sports club. In a physiotherapist's rooms, short-wave diathermy and ultrasound are used to penetrate the tissues more deeply and produce an increase in temperature of up to 5 or 6°C to a depth of 5 cm. This increases the blood flow even more, and the heat can reach more blood vessels.

Muscular work or exercise can increase the amount of heat produced in a muscle to ten or twenty times that in the same muscle at rest.

Age of the patient

There are 'natural delays' in the healing of older individuals. It takes almost twice as long for a wound to close completely in a 40-year-old man as it does in one of 20. Similarly, the tearing strength of wounds (scars) in older people is significantly lower than that in young people. Younger individuals have an earlier and greater increase in metabolism (the supply of energy), allowing for faster healing rates. Further observations suggest that, although the amount of collagen in a wound is similar in old and young patients, the rate of turnover is higher in the young. This would increase remodelling and give greater strength per unit of collagen. As we age, the maximum tensile strength in the elastic modules of collagen decreases. The rate of adaptation to stress is slower with increasing age.

The net clinical result of these changes in an older athlete is a marked increase in the healing time and increases in over-use syndromes and fatigue failures in muscles and tendons.

Steroids

Steroid drugs have an adverse effect on collagen and wound healing. Impairment of wound strength by cortisone was first reported in 1950, and has since been confirmed in numerous clinical studies. Both cortisone and methylprednisolone retard collagen accumulation in experimental granulation tissue during the first two weeks of healing. Generally, hydrocortisone should not be injected into the weight-bearing tissues of an athlete's lower limb.

As anyone who does not play sport regularly will generally rest after an injury, and cortisone does help to relieve pain and inflammation, non-athletes can usually tolerate steroid injections with no noticeable immediate ill effects. But, because of the natural weakening effect of cortisone on healing (and other) tissues, people tempted to overload the injured structure too soon will suffer more damage.

Steroid injections are banned in the treatment of racehorses and greyhounds, yet medical practitioners still give them to humans. If your medical practitioner is adamant that steroids should be used to treat your condition – or that of your patient – it is important to establish that they understand the true, long-term effects of such treatments, and to establish the number of times that they have performed such an injection. The use of steroids in sport has other, more pertinent implications.

Immobilisation

Immobilisation of damaged tissue has many negative effects. The rate of the return of function of muscle, tendon, bone and fibrous tissue have been well studied. These effects are discussed further later in this chapter (page 39).

Activity and exercise

Regular, cyclic, loading increases strength of connective tissues. Because of the natural weakness of healing scar tissue, there are many positive desirable effects to be gained by controlled exercise. Similarly, because of the contractile nature of the scar tissue, controlled stretching exercises can re-orient and restructure the tissues to a more functional level.

Tension and pressure on the growing collagen fibres will determine the direction in which they will lie and, if space permits, their numbers. Fibres therefore develop along the lines of tension. Mild tension enhances tensile strength but too much tension can be disruptive and undesirable. Repeated forceful stretching of ligament and capsular tissues will tend to increase the inflammation, resulting in more scar tissue formation and, more seriously, will continue to impair the flexibility and elasticity.

Exercise also increases blood supply to the injured area, which can enhance the healing effect. The advantages of exercise over heat application in this context are discussed in Chapter 6.

> ## REMEMBER
> *Mild tension enhances tensile strength*

Nerve damage

Damage to sections of the nerves supplying skin, connective tissue and muscle does not alter the rate or quality of healing. Acute **denervation** has no effect on wound healing as long as the damaged point is not under stress.

> **denervation**
> *cutting of or interfering with nerve supply, by damage, disease or drugs*

Size of wound

Epithelium, connective tissue and vessels each grow at a uniform rate throughout the healing period. The initial size of the wound does not affect their rate of growth.

Oedema (swelling)

Moderate oedema has little or no effect on the wound's gain of tensile strength. However, marked oedema has a slight and temporary inhibitory effect on healing. This effect may be more mechanical than biochemical in nature. It is therefore important to keep swelling to a minimum at all stages of rehabilitation.

PROGRESS CHECK   Can you identify four factors that might affect the quality of wound healing?

Healing of specific tissues

Skin

Wound healing is a complex process involving cell movement. The pattern of wound repair is different in different individuals, with different skin types.

Epithelialisation is retarded by the dry scab which normally covers a superficial wound. If the formation of a scab is prevented by keeping the wound moist (and scrupulously clean), the rate of epithelialisation is markedly increased.

> **epithelialisation**
> *formation of epithelium*

Cartilage

Cartilage possesses restricted powers of regeneration. Wounds in cartilage heal by the formation of fibrous scars, around which cartilage cells divide and in time replace the scar tissue. Regeneration is a slow process, lasting many weeks, and apparently varies greatly in different types of cartilage. This is particularly obvious in the rib cartilages, which may take months to heal.

Most cartilage types, though relatively non-vascular, are penetrated by numerous small canals, each conveying a small artery and vein. However, articular hyaline cartilage (the most prominent being the meniscus of the knee) has very few blood vessels through it. It derives its nutrients from the vessels of the synovial membrane, the synovial fluid and the blood vessels of the underlying marrow cavity. If this structure is damaged it will not regenerate. If it is surgically removed, new fibrocartilage will replace it but the new cartilage is not of the same quality, shape and structure as the original articular cartilage.

Tendons and ligaments

These are formed in response to tensile strains in situations where strength is required without rigidity or extensibility.

When a tendon or ligament is severed or partly injured, fibroblasts grow in from the surrounding connective tissue and arrange themselves on strands of fibrin, which form during inflammation induced by the injury and extend from one stump to the other. The fibroblasts become elongated and form collagen fibres which (as usual) are at first fine and gradually become thicker.

The blood supply to tendons and ligaments is poor so healing is slow, much slower than more copiously supplied tissue such as muscle.

The parallel alignment of fibres in a tendon and their orientation along the direction of maximum tension exerted by associated muscle suggests that tension over the region of regeneration will determine the structure of the new tissue.

Muscle

The repair of damage to skeletal muscle involves two separate processes – the formation of non-contractile collagenous fibres and muscle regeneration.

Following injury, the tissue is infiltrated by macrophages. These cells are converted to fibroblasts, which proliferate rapidly in the damaged area. The fibroblasts secrete a soluble protein precursor of collagen and, in their mature form, the cells remain in the tissue as fibrocytes. The process of maturation is accompanied by a shortening of the fibrocytes, leading to the tendency of muscle wounds to heal short.

The biological key to healing of muscles is the knowledge that muscle cells regenerate. In experimental work with total muscle ruptures functional regrowth and regenerating muscle occurred but complete recovery (in terms of strength) was not achieved. The new muscle contained relatively few fibres and large amounts of connective tissue, so the total tension that the muscle was able to produce was less than that of normal muscle. Fortunately, sporting injuries are rarely this severe. However, the same procedure (with the same limitations) will take place in varying degrees depending on the amount of damage to the muscle or its component structures.

A serious complication of muscle injuries during healing is myositis ossificans. This **ossification** process is caused by osteoblasts (cells that form bone) invading the **haematoma** formed at the time of the injury. The osteoblasts are probably derived from the damaged periosteum (the outer coating of bone). Maturation of these cells in the muscle leads to the formation of an open network of bone. If this is not properly managed it can seriously impair future function.

ossification
formation of bone

haematoma
a swelling composed of blood

PROGRESS CHECK Explain the healing capacity of the following: skin, cartilage, tendon, ligament, muscle.

Scar tissue and patient management

Damage to soft tissue in the human body is repaired by non-specific connective tissue, which is composed very largely of the fibrous protein collagen. Basically the same type of connective scar tissue develops at the end of healing – irrespective of the tissue injured, whether it be skin, tendon, ligament or muscle.

Scar tissue is diminished in many of the fitness parameters of the tissue that it is replacing, particularly the two important components of flexibility and strength. Other constituents of fitness, such as agility, co-ordination, endurance, speed and power will be affected to varying degrees, and an athlete returning from injury may be disadvantaged in skills requiring these facilities.

Management of rigidity and loss of extensibility of scar tissue

One of the drawbacks of scar tissue is its rigidity and tendency to contract and deform. Bioengineers have shown that extensibility is as important functionally as strength – for a muscle to attain its full power it must be fully stretched before contraction. Many workers have drawn attention to the fact that fibrosis and scarring in muscle injuries leads to tethering and functional shortening. It has also been claimed that if a muscle is kept in a shortened or relaxed position when healing the resultant scar tissue will form a short bridge, which may tear again when the muscle is fully stretched out for the first time.

It is therefore important that stretching exercises are started early if normal flexibility is to be regained. For example, by careful active stretching of haematomas (bruises) as far as possible before experiencing pain

- **adhesion** formation was limited
- the thigh muscles were able to return to the pre-injury range of motion.

This principle is supported by research which has noted that pressure and tension improve contraction caused by scarring.

The essence of all active treatment of muscle injuries in trained athletes is that active rehabilitation of the muscle can be commenced during healing. In other words, one does not need to wait for full anatomical healing before starting to retrain the muscle. Retraining can be started – gradually at first – during the healing period.

The same principle also applies to injuries of ligaments and tendons. For example, unless exercises are commenced to gradually restore the full range of movement after an injury to the ankle joint, a chronic sprained ankle may result – with associated pain, swelling and movement limitations.

This principle is substantiated by the physiological healing process itself. Collagen fibres, which after injury may form a random mesh, coiled and kinked, cannot contract – but they can be stretched. Stretching is merely a straightening reorientation of the fibres, without changing their dimensions.

> **adhesion**
> *union of normally separate parts by new tissue, produced as a result of inflammation*

PROGRESS CHECK

If the extensibility of scar tissue is as important, functionally, as its strength, how would you manage an injured ligament?

The most important way of controlling contraction is by performing a range of carefully planned movement exercises, which help to remodel the developing collagen. Since there is a high collagen turnover in new wounds, properly applied physical therapy can remodel the scar tissue. Range of motion exercises ignore contraction due to fibroblast pull and concentrate on remodelling the collagen as it is laid down.

It is important that exercises are carried out within limits of pain. **Whatever hurts is wrong; whatever does not hurt is right.** *Pain is nature's guideline, and if stretching exercises are pushed too far into the painful range more soft tissue damage may result – leading to further scar formation.*

The best way to permanently lengthen connective tissue structures, including scar formations, without compromising their structural integrity is to use prolonged, low-intensity stretching at elevated tissue temperatures, cooling the tissue before releasing the tension.

Tensile strength of scar tissue

Collagen has an important role in the strength of wounds. Collagen is the substance used when the body requires tensile strength. Thus tendons and ligaments are composed largely of collagen, and liver and muscle have a lower collagen content.

As discussed in Chapter 2, there are several types of collagen. In this chapter the following are important:

- type I collagen is mostly found in skin, bone and tendon
- type II collagen is the major form in cartilage
- type III is found in scar tissue and in the walls of the blood vessels, intestine and uterus.

pathogenesis
development of disease

Although the collagen in tendons is normally type I, it is replaced by the more flexible type III collagen during repair. Other studies suggest that type III collagen may form a scaffolding in early dermal wound healing but is later replaced by type I collagen. Such alterations in collagen types may be extremely important in normal healing and in **pathogenesis** of abnormal wound repair.

REMEMBER

Scar tissue is never as strong as the tissue it replaces.

Cross-linking and remodelling of collagen fibres may take between 6 months and a year to complete (the longer time being observed in essentially fibrous tissue such as fascia) and it is important to appreciate that the apparently well healed wound is still a weak and brittle structure five months after injury. Tensile strength at that time is known to be only about 10% of the normal value.

The ability of a wound to resist rupture should be assessed from its energy absorption capabilities:

- after 10 days, a wound has recovered 4% of its unwounded value
- after 150 days, it has recovered only just over 50% of its original value.

To compensate for the lack of strength in scar tissue, the athlete should follow an intensive, well planned strengthening programme. When the injury has occurred in a musculotendinous unit, the athlete undergoes a training programme to develop strength, power and endurance. Similarly, following injury to a joint the damaged structures and the muscles controlling the joint must be strengthened. Clinical observation and experimental evidence show that overload appears to strengthen ligaments. There is a close relationship between the strength of the knee ligaments and the mechanical stress to which they are subjected. Other workers have found that the ligament strength of people who exercise is greater than those who don't.

The strength of repaired ligaments is increased with exercise training and decreased by immobilisation.

Thus, a tissue is as strong as the load that is placed on it.

PROGRESS CHECK

- Complete the following sentence: whatever hurts is ———, whatever does not is ———.
- What is the best way to lengthen connective tissue structures?
- What are tendons and ligaments largely composed of?
- Is scar tissue as strong as the tissue it replaces?
- When an injury occurs in a musculotendinous unit, what does the athlete need to develop?

KEY TERMS

You need to know what these words mean. Go back through the chapter or check the glossary to find out.

Healing	Remodelling	Intra
Inflammation	Vascularised	Inter

4 First aid and the management of the injured athlete

After working through this chapter you will be able to:
- ➤ describe the immediate procedure for on-site management of the injured athlete
- ➤ recognise the initial signs of soft-tissue injury
- ➤ implement the appropriate treatment methods at this acute stage
- ➤ understand the uses of ice, compression, elevation and rest
- ➤ demonstrate the use of bandaging and strapping as appropriate.

Although this chapter will look at the immediate management of injury at the site of the activity, it will only outline procedures. It is of vital importance for every person responsible for the medical/therapeutic welfare of any athlete to be a qualified first aider – to hold a recognised qualification from the St John Ambulance, the Red Cross or the Health and Safety Executive.

What you will read in this chapter is over and above what you should already know as a qualified first aider. You should already be capable of dealing with:

- unconsciousness (ABC)
- spinal injuries
- fractures
- bleeding
- shock
- heat injuries
- cramps
- kicks in the abdomen or testicles
- head and facial injuries
- skin injuries (cuts, abrasions, grass burns and blisters).

On-site management

Probably the most difficult part of injury prevention is encountered by the first aider called to attend a player/athlete who has sustained an injury. The first aider must decide whether or not the athlete should retire from that game/sport. You need a methodical system to manage injuries on the field: follow the procedure taught to you during your training as a first aider. An example of such a procedure is PALM.

PALM

This is a mnemonic:

P   avoid **p**anic
A   **a**ssess, then **a**sk, (or ABC)
L   **l**ook (without manhandling)
M   test **m**ovement.

Avoid panic

The most important single thing to remember in the emergency situation is not to panic. Hurry to the injured athlete, but don't be pressured into a hasty decision by an excited crowd, a frustrated athlete or an over-enthusiastic referee.

A calm, accurate assessment of the situation can avoid an athlete's premature removal from the event, or may prevent them from continuing with an injury that could seriously be worsened by further exercise. So – do not panic.

Assess, Ask or ABC

On reaching the injured athlete, quickly assess the situation. If they are unconscious, remember the ABC – check **a**irways, **b**reathing and **c**irculation. An unconscious athlete should be seen by a doctor, if possible, before being moved.

If the athlete is conscious, and the problem is not immediately obvious (such as a dislocated shoulder), ask what is the matter, but do not immediately touch the injured area. Do not drag the athlete to their feet before anything else is done – this could have disastrous results. If the athlete is not sure exactly what happened, ask someone else – the referee, other athletes or even bystanders. Ask leading questions to help gain an accurate picture of the history. This can be a tremendous help in formulating a diagnosis and thereby guiding your decision making.

For example, if a footballer has hurt an ankle, ask:

- Did they fall?
- Were they kicked?
- Did they hear or feel a crack?
- Were they moving?
- If so, in what direction?
- How did they fall?

Such questions will help you to reach a positive diagnosis.

Look without manhandling

You can further assess the extent of the injury simply by looking at it. Signs that will help to localise and identify the condition include swelling, bleeding, abnormal deviations of limbs, the colour of the patient and the injured area, and the position the athlete was in when you arrived.

If the injured area is swollen at this early examination, it is an indication of rapid tissue bleeding – swelling in normal inflammatory processes takes up to two hours to become obvious. If the injured limb has turned white or pale, it is an indication of arterial blockage; if it changes to blue, the

---

REMEMBER

As a first aider, your initial role is purely to find out what is wrong. If the athlete is able to continue by their own efforts, no treatment should be necessary. The application of the 'magic sponge' that we see all too often serves only to refresh players and to give them a breather. However, this, coupled with the knowledge that their injury isn't serious, helps the injured player make a remarkable recovery.

venous circulation is probably impeded or blocked. Any of these conditions will generally necessitate immediate removal from the activity.

Test movement

The athlete should first test movement in the injured area – then you do this. Injured athletes should be encouraged to remain quiet until they have demonstrated their ability to move all limbs unassisted. Nothing which tends to increase pain should be done, as it almost certainly will increase the damage. If the patient can move all their limbs comfortably, they can be encouraged to stand – by their own efforts. If the athlete has to be helped to his or her feet they are not going to get back into the game or activity, and may damage themselves further by attempting to do so.

REMEMBER

*First the athlete moves, then you move – **never** the other way round.*

PROGRESS CHECK

- What first aid qualification do you have or are you taking?
- What does the mnemonic PALM stand for?

If the athlete cannot move the injured limb unassisted, gently try to move it yourself to find what may be limiting the motion. If this increases the athlete's pain, he or she should be brought from the field to a place where a more searching examination can take place.

If the athlete has to be removed from the field, active treatment should be started immediately. Treatment may consist of applying emergency procedures or following the techniques suggested later in this chapter for immediate management of soft-tissue injury.

GOOD PRACTICE ▷ *In managing injuries at the track or on the field, bear in mind the four points contained in the mnemonic PALM:*

- *avoid **p**anic*
- ***a**ssess the situation, then ask about the problem or apply the **ABC***
- ***l**ook but don't manhandle*
- *test **m**ovement – the injured person himself, then you.*

Immediate treatment of soft-tissue injuries

It must be stressed that speed in applying an active, proven treatment to an injury is one of the most important factors in quick healing. This, of course, applies to all categories of injuries. However, this section deals only with soft-tissue injuries and their first aid management. In this context, soft tissue refers to ligaments, muscles, tendons, fascia (fibrous tissue), and similar structures. Most sporting injuries involve injuries to soft tissues.

The usual signs of tissue reaction to injury are:

- inflammation
- bleeding

- swelling
- loss of function
- pain
- muscle spasm.

The important aim in the early stages of treatment is to minimise these effects to speed healing and eventual return to sport. Efforts should be directed at preventing and reducing inflammation, stopping the bleeding and relieving pain and spasm. By following the guidelines contained in the mnemonic ICER (**i**ce, **c**ompression, **e**levation, **r**est) you will do as much as any person can do, qualified or otherwise.

Ice

Ice is applied to an injury for two main reasons:

1   It reduces the circulation to the area and thus reduces the swelling
2   It is an efficient reliever of pain and muscle spasm.

A full discussion on the effects of ice and its application as a treatment modality appears in Chapter 6.

The normal soft-tissue injury will slowly swell for at least 24 hours because exudates are brought by the circulatory and lymphatic systems as part of the normal healing processes.

The normal clotting mechanism of the blood will generally stop the bleeding within the first five minutes, but the vasoconstrictive effect of ice treatment will help to prevent and control excess swelling regardless of whether the cause is inflammation or bleeding.

However, the most important use of ice at this stage is as an **analgesic**. After five minutes' application, during which the patient feels

analgesic
relieving pain

- cold
- then pain
- then numbness,

the ice elevates the pain threshold, increasing the patient's tolerance to pain. This in turn facilitates early mobilisation of the injured limb.

Ice can be effectively applied in four different ways – ice packs, ice massage, ice baths, ice sprays – but it should *never* be applied directly to the skin, as it can cause skin burns. The most effective temperature range for pain relief is 6–10°C. *Never* use dry ice (frozen carbon dioxide), as its temperature can drop to below –43°C, which would cause extensive skin damage.

GOOD PRACTICE ▷ *Place the injured limb, regardless of the site of injury, in a moist towel containing crushed ice. An injured ankle or wrist may be submerged in a bucket of ice water. Leave in this situation for no more than 15 minutes, and repeat this procedure every two waking hours for 24–48 hours.*

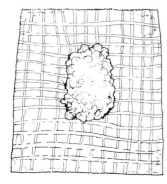

Figure 4.1 *Ice should be wrapped in a towel, never applied directly to the skin*

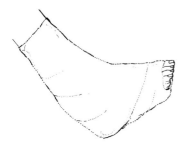

Figure 4.2 *An ice pack wrapped around an injured area will stay cold for about 40 minutes*

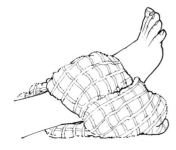

Figure 4.3 *The first layer of the compression bandage: 'cotton wool' or 'gamgee'*

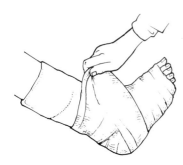

Figure 4.4 *Next apply the crepe bandage covering*

Some books will tell you to leave the ice on the athlete for 20–30 minutes but recent research shows that after 20 minutes the initial effect of the ice (vasoconstriction) is reversed and vasodilation occurs, the effect of which could slow the initial stages of the healing process.

It is unwise to use heat of any description in this phase, because heat can cause bleeding to start again. If ice is applied correctly, following the guidelines above, rebleeding won't occur.

Compression

A crepe bandage comfortably wrapped around the injury also helps to prevent excess swelling (Figures 4.3 and 4.4). However, if the bandage is too tight, or if the fluid is allowed to build up as the limb remains pendant, the bandage may then act as a tourniquet. Keep a check on the extremities for blueness, which indicates lack of circulation, and numbness, which suggests compression of a nerve. If either occurs, loosen the bandage.

Elevation

As the amount of excess fluid at the site of injury is influenced by the force of gravity, keep the injured limb raised, particularly if it is the ankle that is injured. This enables fluid to drain away from the injury, back into the circulatory and lymphatic systems, thus preventing accumulation and eventual scarring in the area.

Rest

With most injuries, 24–48 hours rest from movement will help to prevent aggravation of the damage and relieve symptoms of shock, pain and spasm. The upper limb should generally be immobilised in a sling and the lower limb supported in a compression bandage.

GOOD PRACTICE ▷ A *good technique is to use ice, compression, elevation and rest at the same time.*

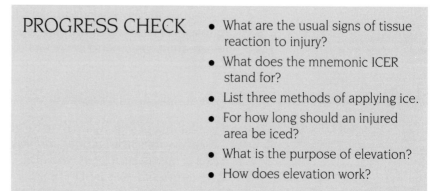

PROGRESS CHECK
- What are the usual signs of tissue reaction to injury?
- What does the mnemonic ICER stand for?
- List three methods of applying ice.
- For how long should an injured area be iced?
- What is the purpose of elevation?
- How does elevation work?

Bandaging and wound dressing

In sports therapy, the main uses of bandages are:

- to protect a wound by covering it with a dressing to maintain hygiene
- to apply compression during the initial stages of an injury in order to control swelling and bleeding
- to restrict movement – such as immobilising a suspected fracture – and thus prevent further injury
- to support a weakened or damaged structure, as in a sling.

Other uses are to support sponge pads under the foot and to secure a protective device over a vulnerable area.

The best dressing for wounds is a sterile melanin dressing.

Principles of bandaging

- Select the appropriate bandage for the job. Rolled bandages are made of many materials: gauze, cotton cloth, crepe and elastic crepe wrapping.
- Choose the correct width for the particular structure – 2 cm for wrist, thumb and hand; 3 cm for ankle and elbow; 6 cm for knee and shoulder; 10 cm for thigh and trunk.
- Hold the bandage with the unrolled portion uppermost and apply the outer surface of the bandage to the injured part.
- Bandage from distal to proximal (from the extremity towards the heart), in the direction of the blood returning to the heart through the veins.
- Unroll only a few centimetres at a time, maintaining even pressure throughout.
- Overlap the bandage by at least half the width of the previous turn.
- Smooth the bandage as it follows the contour of the skin and limb.
- Finish off with a straight turn above the part, fold in the end and fasten.
- Watch for reaction of circulation between the bandage and the extremity. If the bandage is too tight, the circulation and nerve pathways will be impeded. Pink is healthy, but if the extremities turn blue or black, lose their pulse, or become numb or tingling, release the pressure immediately.

Common bandaging techniques

There are many different techniques for bandaging, some of which you will have been taught on your first aid course (Figure 4.5). The secret is to keep things simple.

Circular or simple spiral
This way of bandaging is used when the injured part is of relatively uniform thickness – such as a finger, the trunk or a forearm.

Reverse spiral
This is used to bandage limbs which are funnel-shaped and for which a simple spiral won't work. An example is the calf.

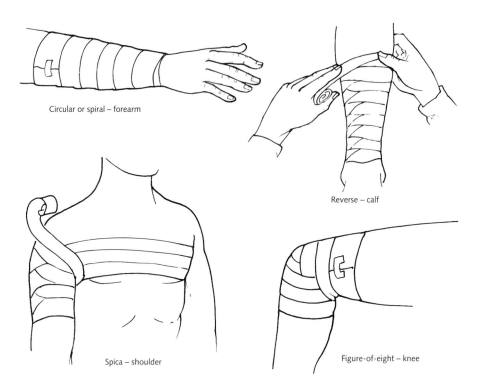

Circular or spiral – forearm

Reverse – calf

Spica – shoulder

Figure-of-eight – knee

Figure 4.5 *Common bandaging techniques*

Figure-of-eight
Use this technique for joints such as the knee, ankle and elbow.

Spica
This is an uneven figure-of-eight used for the thumb, shoulder or hip.

It is always a good idea to keep an adequate record of the 'first aid' management of anyone. You could use a preprinted form like the one shown in Figure 4.6.

PROGRESS CHECK

- What are the main uses of bandages in sports therapy?
- Which structure would you use the following width of bandages for: 2 cm, 3 cm, 6 cm, 10cm?

── KEY TERMS ──

You need to know what these words mean. Go back through the chapter or check the glossary to find out.	Test Ice	Compression Elevation	Rest

1. Name _____ Home address_____

2. Time accident occurred_____ am/pm. Date _____

3. Place of accident: ☐ training ☐ competition ☐ other (specify)

4. *Nature of injury:*

   ☐ abrasion ☐ bite ☐ bruise ☐ burn ☐ concussion ☐ cut

   ☐ dislocation ☐ fracture ☐ laceration ☐ puncture ☐ scalds

   ☐ scratches ☐ shock (electrical) ☐ sprain ☐ other (specify)

   Part of body injured:

   ☐ abdomen ☐ ankle ☐ arm ☐ back ☐ chest ☐ ear ☐ elbow

   ☐ eye ☐ face ☐ finger ☐ foot ☐ hand ☐ head ☐ knee ☐ leg

   ☐ mouth ☐ nose ☐ scalp ☐ tooth ☐ wrist ☐ other (specify)

5. Description of accident:

6. Immediate action taken:

   ☐ first-aid treatment given by [name]: _____

   ☐ sent to doctor by [name] _____

   Doctor's name _____

   ☐ sent to hospital [name]_____

   Hospital name _____

7. Treatment prescribed: ☐ physiotherapy ☐ rest ☐ medication

   ☐ other (specify)

8. Recommended length of lay-off:

9. Was a parent or other individual notified? ☐ yes ☐ no

   When? _____ How? _____

   By whom? [name] _____

   Name of individual notified:_____

10. Witnesses: (1) Name_____Address _____

    (2) Name_____Address _____

11. Remarks:

Figure 4.6 *Sample first aid record form*

5 The consultation process

After working through this chapter you will be able to:

➤ demonstrate a subjective assessment
➤ design an appropriate consultation card
➤ demonstrate an objective assessment
➤ look at and assess posture
➤ use your understanding of range of movement to assess a patient
➤ assess and diagnose accurately

An injured sportsperson wants to get back to their sport as soon as physically possible. The sports therapist therefore must be sure that what they are doing is helping the athlete obtain that goal – get this first consultation wrong and very valuable time can be wasted, the injury could be made worse and the athlete will be far from happy.

In this book the evaluation of the injured athlete will follow the SOAP routine:

S **Subjective** assessment
O **Objective** assessment
A Assessment of information
P Plan treatment.

subjective
based on personal feelings

objective
external to the mind, actual

Before beginning to take the history and starting the physical examination the sports therapist should make every effort to establish a rapport with the athlete, to help him or her feel comfortable and ready to co-operate in therapy.

The patient should be positioned as comfortably as possible. This means that he or she may need to lie down on the couch from the beginning of the examination, or may be more comfortable sitting in a chair.

GOOD PRACTICE ▷ *The sports therapist should help the patient to position the injured parts in the most comfortable position, using pillows, blankets for support or warmth if needed. The temperature of the examination area should be comfortable for all participants. There should be no glare from lights, and the room or cubicle should be private, with doors closed or curtains drawn.*

The therapist should also make sure that any person attending with the patient is also comfortable and close to hand if required. It is sadly sometimes necessary for the therapist to have a third party present when they are with a patient.

Subjective assessment

The sports therapist does this before he or she even touches the athlete. Some basic information should be established:

- start with the obvious things – name, address, telephone number and date of birth
- the patient's physical activities
- the patient's job
- the sport that was involved with this injury
- the types of physical training the athlete participates in
- the symptoms of the injury itself.

Do not try to be clever and guess what is wrong, much as you might wish to.

We really need to understand what our patient is telling us – for example, if they say an injured area aches, what exactly do they mean?

GOOD PRACTICE ▷ *The secret of successful consultation is to ask. If you are unclear about what someone means, ask them to explain. If you try to second guess, you will make mistakes.*

ACTIVITY   Can you think of 50 words that could be used to describe pain?

What should we be asking?

After getting all of the initial information, the therapist needs to move slowly and clearly through a number of appropriate questions. Therapists often use a preprinted consultation card which has on it all the questions they are likely to need to ask. But remember that all injuries are different and that no two patients are the same. It would be ludicrous to go through a whole range of pointless questions with every patient.

GOOD PRACTICE ▷ *Each consultation must be tailored to the individual patient's needs – and, more importantly, to your needs as the therapist. This will enable you to put together a complete and accurate picture of the patient, their condition and their lifestyle.*

Questions that you might care to use as and when appropriate are:

- What is the patient's chief complaint?
- When did it begin – was it of sudden or slow onset?
- Has the problem been continuous or is it intermittent?
- Has this problem occurred before?
- Did a traumatic incident occur before the present condition?
- What are the present symptoms?
- If there is pain – what kind of pain is it?
- What makes the condition feel better or worse?
- Did the part injured change colour? If so, when and for how long?
- Has the patient seen their doctor or any other therapist?
- Were any X-rays taken?

The sports therapist must understand and be able to justify why he or she is asking any question. Remember that a patient might just ask why you wish to know something.

What should the consultation notes look like?

You should design a consultation card that is suitable for your needs. Once you have gained experience, you may find preprinted cards that restrict the space available for comment very frustrating. When designing your card, remember:

- what you need to know
- how much room you need
- that the notes should be updated every time you see your patient.

An example of such a card is given in Figure 5.1. This card will be used throughout the chapter to illustrate important points.

Differential diagnosis

Pinpointing areas of concern

Once you have the basic information you need, you must narrow down the areas of concern and the structures that might be causing the problem.

You should produce a complete listing for each area of the body. The example that follows covers the lower limb.

GOOD PRACTICE ▷ *The best way of doing this is to produce a number of charts for you to use until you become familiar with all of the muscles/joints/tendon/ligaments and conditions that might be involved. These are known as differential diagnosis cards.*

SPORTS THERAPY CLINIC
CONSULTATION CARD

Name .... **Date of Birth** ....

Address... **Telephone Number** ....

.... **Work Number**..

.... **Doctor** ....

.... **Telephone**..

Patient Complaint:

History/Subjective Assessment:

Date of Consultation: _____

Objective Assessment:

Diagnosis:

Treatment Plan:

Figure 5.1 *Sample blank consultation card*

SPORTS THERAPY CLINIC
DIFFERENTIAL DIAGNOSIS

Joints/Muscles of the lower limb

Joints	Muscles

Joints	Muscles
Hip Knee Ankle	Rectus femoris Vastus lateralis Vastus medialis Vastus intermedius Sartorius Adductor magnus Adductor longus Adductor brevis Biceps femoris Semitendinosus Semimembranosus Gracilis Gastrocnemius Tibialis anterior Peroneus longus Flexor digitorum longus Extensor digitorum longus Achilles tendon Soleus

Patient's Name:
Address:
Telephone Number:

Figure 5.2   *Diagnosis chart for the lower limb*

Only once the areas of concern have been narrowed down is it appropriate to commence the objective assessment.

PROGRESS CHECK

- What information should you obtain from every patient?
- What other information would you like to know?

Objective physical assessment

This section consists of points to look for when examining the whole body – but clearly you should use only the tests that are appropriate to your patient's injury.

Equipment needed for examining musculoskeletal and other tissues:

- scales
- percussion hammer
- goniometer
- orange sticks
- cotton wool
- tape measure.

The following principles should be observed when performing the objective/physical examination.

- Examine the normal (uninvolved) tissues before injured, inflamed or otherwise involved tissues.
- **Bilateral** observations must always be made for comparison.
- Local (site-specific) signs and symptoms are compared with **systemic** findings.
- **Palpation** is done gently, while observing facial and other responses to note sensitivity or tenderness within tissues.
- Movements are assessed within normal ranges of movements.
- Comparisons should be made with the uninjured parts in the same position.
- Inspection (observation) always includes looking at both sides of the patient for:
  - shape, contour, size and symmetry
  - signs of inflammation (heat or hot areas, colour changes, swelling, pain, tenderness or soreness)
  - bruises or discoloured areas
  - muscle fullness, **hypertrophy** or **atrophy**
  - deformity.

The steps of the musculoskeletal examination should follow this pattern:

- inspection
- **auscultation**
- palpation
- range of motion measurements (active movements are performed before passive movement) and joint play
- measurements of muscle strength
- reflex testing (if appropriate).

All findings should be documented completely after the examination. Always compare the findings with what is considered normal.

The patient can be examined while standing, sitting or lying down. First observe the body's alignment and stature. Then look for:

---

bilateral
two sided, on both sides

systemic
affecting the entire body or organism

palpation
examination by touch

hypertrophy
abnormal enlargement of an organ or tissue

atrophy
wasting away

---

auscultation
examination by listening

- obvious deformities
- spinal curvatures
- hypertrophied or atrophied limbs
- size of body and stature related to age and sex
- scars, marks, masses and skin openings.

| **gait** |
| *manner of walking* |

Initial observations of **gait**, posture, stature, and gross abnormalities may be made as the patient enters the room while clothed. For the rest of the examination, the patient should be positioned with their joints in the position of greatest stability for comfort.

Normal findings

Posture

Normal posture is shown in Figure 5.3. In the normal, uninjured patient

- posture is upright and erect
- the head is in the midline and perpendicular to shoulders and spinal column
- the shoulders and pelvis are aligned
- the arms hang freely from the shoulders
- feet are planted firmly on the floor with the toes pointing straight ahead
- there is a concave curve to the cervical and lumbar spines
- the thoracic spine has a convex curve.

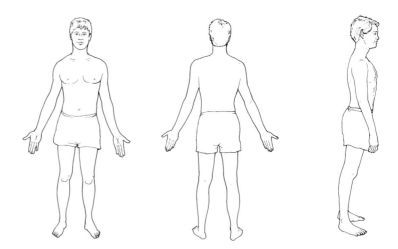

Figure 5.3 *The body posture should be examined from the front, back and side*

Stature
This should be normal for age and sex according to actuarial tables.

Symmetry
The two sides should appear equal but may be slightly different because of handedness.

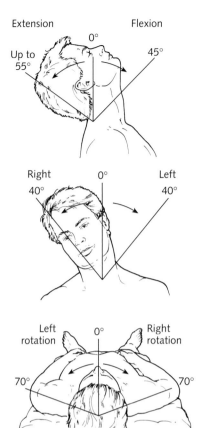

Figure 5.4 *Range of motion of the cervical spine*

Gait

Gait should be easy and rhythmic, with steps about 30-45 cm in length and normal heel–toe placement. Stride is without hitch, lurch, sway or tilt. Arms should swing freely, and the patient is balanced and erect through each phase of walking away, turning, and returning. As the patient turns, the head and face should turn before the rest of the body.

The older adult

In an older person the following variations are normal:

- posture is less upright and erect
- head and neck may be more forward
- shoulders may be rolled or hunched forward
- feet may be closer together or farther apart (especially in women), with the angle of the feet and legs decreased at hip area, leading to varus placement of legs and feet
- the upper extremities appear longer and out of proportion to rest of the body.

The patient is slower to initiate and stop walking. He or she may shuffle at times, with less ankle and knee lifting. Steps are shorter, more rapid and less rhythmic.

Variations

Using the guidelines in Figures 5.4–5.11, you should be able to form a clear picture of normal findings – what you would expect – and variations from normal – what you actually find.

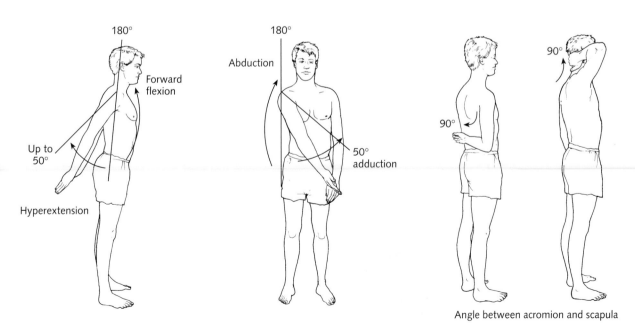

Figure 5.5 *Range of motion of the shoulder*

Hyperextension

Flexion

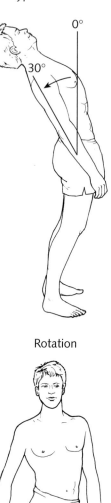

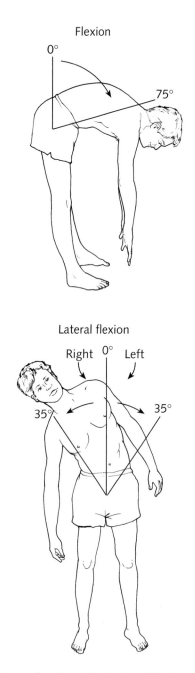

Lateral flexion

Rotation

Figure 5.6   *Range of motion of the thoracic and lumbar spine*

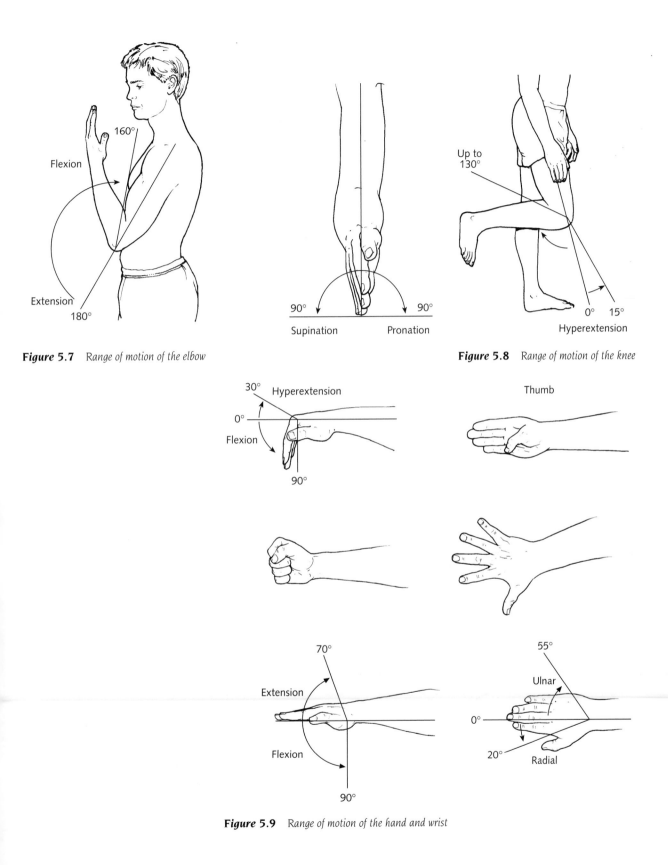

Figure 5.7   *Range of motion of the elbow*

Figure 5.8   *Range of motion of the knee*

Figure 5.9   *Range of motion of the hand and wrist*

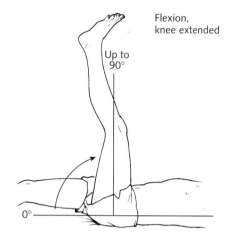

Flexion,
knee extended

Up to
90°

0°

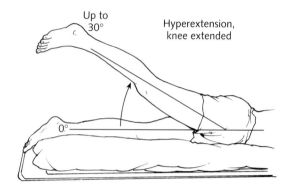

Up to
30°

Hyperextension,
knee extended

0°

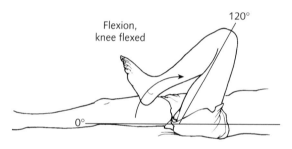

Flexion,
knee flexed

120°

0°

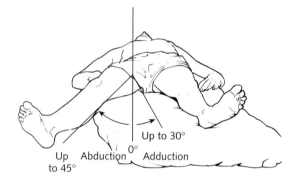

Up to 30°

Up
to 45°

Abduction

0°

Adduction

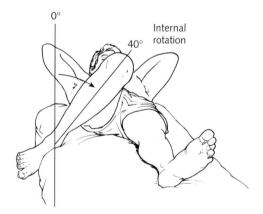

0°

40°

Internal
rotation

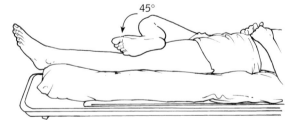

45°

Figure 5.10 *Range of motion of the hip*

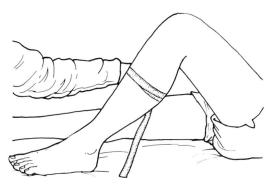

Widest part of calf

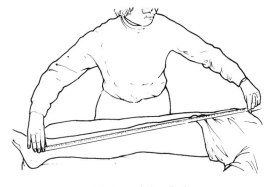

Hip to medial malleolus

Figure 5.11   *Measuring leg dimensions*

Knowledge of the range of motion is an important tool – write it down, put it up on the wall, do whatever you have to do to help you remember.

GOOD PRACTICE ▷ *If you work regularly with particular athletes or a team, keep records of their range of movements to enable you to accurately identify any problems.*

You should now go back to your differential diagnosis sheet and tick off anything that you have been able to rule out.

Assessment of information

At the end of each stage of the consultation process you must assess the information you have obtained. Always follow the same routine, using the appropriate differential diagnosis assessment card:

- question subjectively
- amend card, deleting uninjured structures
- assess objectively – look at the structures remaining on your card, remembering always to look at the uninjured area first and then compare with the injured side
- amend the card further, deleting each structure as it is checked and injury discounted
- make the diagnosis – you should now be left with an accurate diagnosis, your card showing only the structure(s) injured.

SPORTS THERAPY CLINIC
DIFFERENTIAL DIAGNOSIS

Joints/Muscles of the lower limb

Joints	Muscles

Joints	Muscles
~~Hip~~ ~~Knee~~ ~~Ankle~~ *(No joint injury)*	Rectus femoris ~~Vastus lateralis~~ ~~Vastus medialis~~ ~~Vastus intermedius~~ ~~Sartorius~~ ~~Adductor magnus~~ ~~Adductor longus~~ ~~Adductor brevis~~ ~~Biceps femoris~~ ~~Semitendinosus~~ ~~Semimembranosus~~ ~~Gracilis~~ ~~Gastrocnemius~~ ~~Tibialis anterior~~ ~~Peroneus longus~~ ~~Flexor digitorum longus~~ ~~Extensor digitorum longus~~ ~~Achilles tendon~~ ~~Soleus~~

Patient's Name:	*Steve Jones*
Address:	*The Club, Woking Rd, Greasby* *Wirrall*
Telephone Number:	*0151-611 3000*

Figure 5.12   *Part-diagnosis chart completed*

SPORTS THERAPY CLINIC
DIFFERENTIAL DIAGNOSIS

Joints/Muscles of the lower limb

Joints	Muscles

Joints	Muscles
~~Hip~~	Rectus femoris *
~~Knee~~	~~Vastus lateralis~~
~~Ankle~~	~~Vastus medialis~~
	~~Vastus intermedius~~
(No joint injury)	~~Sartorius~~
	~~Adductor magnus~~
	~~Adductor longus~~
	~~Adductor brevis~~
	~~Biceps femoris~~
	~~Semitendinosus~~
	~~Semimembranosus~~
	~~Gracilis~~
	~~Gastrocnemius~~
	~~Tibialis anterior~~
	~~Peroneus longus~~
	~~Flexor digitorum longus~~
	~~Extensor digitorum longus~~
	~~Achilles tendon~~
	~~Soleus~~

Patient's Name:	*Steve Jones*
Address:	*The Club, Woking Rd, Greasby Wirrall*
Telephone Number:	*0151-611 3000*

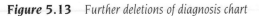

Figure 5.13 *Further deletions of diagnosis chart*

SPORTS THERAPY CLINIC
CONSULTATION CARD

Name Steve Jones

Address The Club

Woking Rd

Greasby

Wirrall

Date of Birth 1 - 2 - 68

Telephone Number 0151-611-3000

Work Number

Doctor Dr. Davies

Telephone 0151-621-1111

Patient Complaint:

Pain in front of (R) thigh

History/Subjective Assessment:

Playing football, felt muscle tighten, very uncomfortable, although continued 24 hours later – very painful, even to walk – No bruising. No contact

Date of Consultation: 7.3.96

Objective Assessment:

No obvious abnormality.

No discoloration.

Restricted contraction of Rect Fem. (R)

Pain recreated on kicking.

Diagnosis:

Partial tear of right rectus femoris.

Treatment Plan:

Relieve pain, strengthen healing scar. Rehabilitate.

Figure 5.14 *The completed consultation card, showing the diagnosis*

Planning treatment

Once you have a diagnosis, you must implement the appropriate treatment. This is discussed at some length in the next chapter.

ACTIVITY

- With a partner demonstrate on each other the full range of movement available in each of the following: cervical spine and neck, thoracic and lumbar spine, shoulders, elbow, wrist, hand and fingers, hips, knees.
- Demonstrate each of the measurement dimensions.

KEY TERMS

You need to know what these words mean. Go back through the chapter or check the glossary to find out.

Subjective	Differential	Palpation
Objective	diagnosis	Posture

6 Methods of treatment and rehabilitation

After working through this chapter you will be able to:

➤ explain the importance of treatment and rehabilitation
➤ demonstrate methods of relieving pain
➤ demonstrate techniques used in the reduction of swelling and relaxation of muscle spasm
➤ demonstrate an understanding of the components of fitness in the area of injury rehabilitation
➤ appreciate the role of flexibility, strength, power, endurance and co-ordination
➤ show a practical understanding of rehabilitation programming and the reinstating of functional activity.

There is often some confusion in the area of treatment and rehabilitation, and more often than not the two areas are separated – but treatment and rehabilitation are one and the same thing. Rehabilitation begins immediately after injury and should continue until the patient is functionally fit and ready to return to their sport. Full functional fitness should be restored as soon as possible – this should be the aim in treatment and rehabilitation of the injured athlete.

We will discuss the methods of treatment and the principles of rehabilitation under three headings:

1 Relief of symptoms – the selection of correct treatments to aid the relief of pain, reduction of swelling and relaxation of any muscle spasm.

2 Regaining the components of fitness of the injured area – selection of therapeutic exercise to aid with flexibility, strength, power, endurance and co-ordination.

3 Regaining functional activity – reinforcing the need to develop a 'treat and train' attitude when treating athletes.

In order to proceed effectively with treatment and rehabilitation we need to control pain, swelling and (if present) any muscle spasm. If we can correctly manage these reactions to the injury we have followed the 'healing process' route and the patient will be able to start with their therapeutic rehabilitation/exercise programme.

In earlier chapters we looked at the immediate treatment (up to the first 48 hours) of injury.

> **REMEMBER**
>
> *It is of vital importance to relieve the pain and any associated muscle spasm and then to reduce any swelling present at the injury site. The ICER regimen is the very best way of achieving this.*

Relief of swelling

As swelling is largely caused by the inability of the blood vessels to contain the extra white blood cells and plasma proteins which accumulate at the injury site, the two most effective ways to manage excess swelling are by compression and elevation, as we have already discussed. The amount of swelling at an injury will depend on:

- the extent of the damage and
- the levels of tension in the surrounding tissues.

For example, a deep muscle injury might not swell as much as one closer to the surface because tension exerted by the skin is weaker than that exerted by deep muscles.

The amount of swelling is also influenced by gravity. If a limb is hanging, fluid (including blood) will accumulate in the area of the wound, or might drop down further. The excess fluid and blood are normally removed by the venous and lymphatic systems of the body. The venous system relies on the pumping action of the surrounding muscles to shunt the fluid back to the heart and then to the liver, where it is broken down and redirected. However, if pain and spasm prevent this muscular action, the fluid will accumulate where the force of gravity dictates. Elevation will therefore play an important part in controlling this swelling, and the injured limb should be raised above the heart wherever possible. A compression bandage will also help to prevent swelling.

Ice is also valuable in the treatment of swelling. As discussed earlier, ice is mainly used for its analgesic effect and because it will prevent fresh bleeding in the early stage of treatment. It should be your first choice over any other form of treatment that also offers pain and spasm relief.

In these early stages there is also a place for non-heat-producing electromedical modalities such as transcutaneous electrical nerve stimulation (TENS), pulsed ultrasound therapy or acupressure point stimulation.

REMEMBER

Heat therapies, including massage, are not recommended in the first 24-48 hours after an injury while the damaged circulatory system is healing and unstable and there is a risk of further bleeding.

PROGRESS CHECK

- What causes swelling?
- The amount of swelling will depend on two things. What are they?
- How is the excess fluid normally removed?

Pain relief

organic
derived from living organisms

psychic
in the mind

Before discussing methods of pain relief, it is necessary to examine the phenomenon of pain itself. The perception of pain is both a physiological and a psychological process which involves receptors, conductors and integrative cerebral mechanisms. The problem of pain assessment is complicated because it is difficult to differentiate **organic** from **psychic** factors, both of which contribute to the final expression of pain.

For these reasons, the patient's perception of pain is not always proportional to the actual structural and functional damage that has occurred, and could delay a positive treatment/rehabilitation programme.

The immediate aim of pain relief is to relieve the sensation of pain enough to make the patient comfortable and able to tolerate movement.

There are many ways to modulate pain perception and, in particular, to elevate the pain threshold.

Cryotherapy

Cryotherapy is the application of cold for therapeutic purposes. The use of cold therapy is well established – it was used by ancient Greek physicians to treat acute injuries and it was also used during the Middle Ages and during the Napoleonic wars as preparative anaesthesia. Because of its long history and general acceptance, a great many different opinions have surrounded its use, and the aims of application are not often understood.

hypothermia
subnormal body temperature

hypoxia
oxygen deficiency

The physiological effects of **hypothermia** are many – and, because of the lack of scientific research, there are several conflicting aspects which need to be looked at. However, for the sports therapist, several facts are now clear. Cryotherapy can be effectively used to treat injury by:

- easing pain in the acute (and later) stages of injury (pain relief)
- reducing secondary **hypoxia**, oedema and bleeding (effect on circulation)
- providing an effective technique for rehabilitation (cryokinetics).

Pain relief
This is perhaps the most important effect of ice during treatment/rehabilitation. Applying ice to the skin produces a sensation of cold, which lasts several minutes. A burning, stinging sensation is then felt (this lasts about 5 minutes) then numbness is achieved in the area. This tends to raise the pain threshold (i.e. it relieves the sensation of pain). The effect is maintained for as long as the skin temperature is lowered.

hypertonicity
muscle spasm

efferent nerve
nerve leading away from an organ or limb

endorphins
the body's natural pain inhibitors

As a protective muscular spasm is generally a direct result of pain, the application of ice will also relieve this spasm. The speed of nerve impulses is governed by the temperature of the tissues surrounding the receptor site. Cooling reduces the conductivity of nerves, and the effect is proportional to the diameter of the nerve. The reduced conductivity of nerves lessens the sensitivity of the muscle spindle and muscle **hypertonicity** is reduced.

Ice also has a counter-irritant effect – the cold receptors respond to cooling by a sharp but transient increase in discharge. This bombards the **efferent nerve** pathways, preventing the sensation of pain reaching the brain.

It is also possible that thermoregulatory defence mechanisms prompt the pituitary gland to release **endorphins** as the cold invades the tissues.

GOOD PRACTICE ▷ *When aiming to reduce pain and spasm, the best temperature is 12–15°C. If aiming to reduce pain only, then 6–12°C can be used.*

Effect on circulation

The initial response to cold is sympathetic vasoconstriction as the body attempts to conserve heat. This consists of:

- direct constriction of the superficial blood vessels
- immediate general vasoconstriction by reflex action through the central nervous system
- delayed general vasoconstriction caused by the effect on the posterior hypothalamus of cool venous blood returning from cooled skin.

This initial vasoconstriction of the injured superficial blood vessels prevents further bleeding and helps to prevent fluids passing into the tissues, reducing excessive swelling.

Experiments have shown that the application of ice can control swelling and limit the magnitude of injury. Hypothermia reduces the energy needs of cells, reducing the tissue's need for oxygen, and the tissue goes into a state of partial hibernation, which minimises the amount of injury. Hypothermia markedly reduces metabolic activity of the tissue cooled.

If the tissues in an injured area that has escaped destruction by the trauma are not 'put into hibernation' by cold, their need for oxygen may be greater than the injured blood vessels can supply – and they could suffer hypoxic injury. This secondary injury will add cellular debris to the haematoma and increase healing time.

Cold does not appear to reduce the inflammatory response, only to delay it. This obviously helps to lessen congestion also in the first 24–48 hours and allows healing to proceed normally.

Cold causes an initial vasoconstriction, which is followed by vasodilation and increase of blood flow to the area. Some authors claim that this effect occurs below 10°C; others suggest 15°C as the turning point. If the cold application is continued, sudden deep tissue vasodilation, lasting 4–6 minutes, will occur. This 'circulatory rush', which is seen as a thermoregulatory defence against thermal insult, can raise the local temperature sixfold. Vasoconstriction is then re-established, followed 15–30 minutes later by vasodilation. This cyclic process has been termed 'the hunting response'. The general level of the peaks of vasodilation tends to decline but if the patient is kept warm, alternation of vasodilation and vasoconstriction may occur for several hours. However, recent research has shown that it's not as simple as this. Cold-induced vasodilation is a very complex mechanism that occurs in different amounts in different parts of the body. It occurs most readily in those areas of the body that are most prone to frostbite – the fingers, toes, cheeks and ears. However, a temperature of −7°C is not severe enough to cause vasodilation of the ankle, although some workers have demonstrated mild vasodilation in the forearm without prior constriction.

The benefit of this 'hunting response' is to flush debris and exudates from the local area of trauma and enhance healing. But, due to the conflicting evidence, it is not clear that this positive therapeutic benefit is actually achieved. On the other hand, because prolonged cold application has desirable effects in these early stages, it may do some good.

REMEMBER

Cold therapy should not be used on patients who are unconscious, semi-conscious, have collagen diseases or vasoplastic conditions. An ice reaction (ice burn) can be expected in 15 cases out of every 1000.

PROGRESS CHECK

- Define pain.
- What is cryotherapy? How is it used in the treatment of injury?

A *technique for rehabilitation – cryokinetics*

The distinction between cold application for acute injuries and cold application for rehabilitation is an important one. After about 48 hours (when the initial acute reaction has settled down), cold may be applied chiefly for its analgesic effect, which will allow early mobility of the injured area. This can be an effective means of rehabilitation, as a 15-minute superficial application of ice produces relaxation, analgesia and relieves muscle spasms. Heat can then be effectively produced at a deeper level by active movement – this stimulates healing and improves local flexibility and strength.

Caution must be used, however, if the patient is asked to exercise vigorously after 60–85 minutes of cold treatment. Ice lowers deep muscular temperature by as much as 15°C. The flexibility of collagen – one of the most important structural materials in tendons, ligaments, muscles and, particularly, scar tissue – is seriously decreased by cold. On the other hand, heat has the effect of increasing tissue extensibility. Muscle cooling below 20°C delays twitch time and tension during muscle contraction. Neuromuscular transmission at the end plate is decreased at temperatures below 15°C and totally blocked at 5°C. Therefore vigorous stretching techniques may be inefficient or even dangerous after intense icing.

PROGRESS CHECK

Explain the principles of cryotherapy.

Manual therapy

As a sports therapist you will undoubtedly encounter the words massage, manipulation and mobilisation. Manipulation is a physiotherapy and osteopathic skill and needs considerable study. It is therefore beyond the scope of this book.

Massage

Many variants of the basic techniques are taught – but the best technique is the one that works well for you and your patients. You should develop your own style, while still remaining faithful to the principles of the ancient art of massage.

Manual massage is a long-established and effective therapy for the relief of pain, swelling, muscle spasm and restricted movement. Various mechanical methods now complement the traditional manual techniques. The manipulative techniques traditionally classified as massage are:

- palpation
- effleurage
- kneading.

Their use arose from the natural, intuitive, desire to rub a painful injury. Massage is widely used in sports medicine and has much to offer the injured athlete. The therapeutic effects of massage include:

- control of swelling
- increased blood flow
- relief of pain
- relief of muscle spasm.

Massage accelerates inflammatory processes and mobilises contracted fibrous tissue. Massage will also affect muscle tone and cause general relaxation.

Tradition defines massage as 'hand motions practised on the surface of the living body with a therapeutic goal'. Therapeutic massage began in France and many of the names used are in French.

Contraindications to massage are few, but include:

- malignancy
- infection of body fluid
- acute injury
- fragile skin.

Clearly, if someone is undergoing medical treatment, you should get clearance from their doctor before commencing any type of massage.

REMEMBER

The best massage technique is the one that works for you and your patients.

Manual techniques

Effleurage

These are slow, rhythmic, stoking hand movements, moulded to the shape of the skin (Figure 6.1). Effleurage frequently begins and ends a treatment session.

---

distal
furthest away from the centre or midline of the body

proximal
nearest to the centre or midline of the body

The strokes pass from **distal** to **proximal** and parallel to the long axis of the tissue. Gradual compression reduces muscle tone and induces a general state of relaxation that relieves muscle spasm and prepares the patient for more vigorous treatment. Firm pressure accelerates blood and lymph flow, improves tissue drainage and thus reduces recent swelling. Rapid strokes have the opposite effect. These will increase muscle tone and may be useful during the final preparation for competition (pre-event preparation).

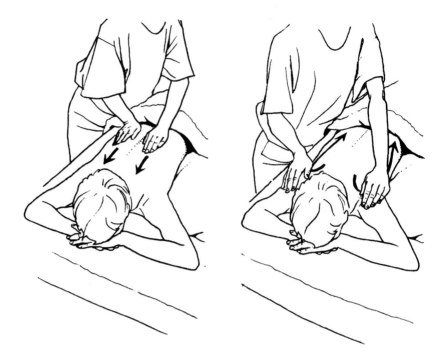

Figure 6.1 *Effleurage*

Kneading

Kneading (Figure 6.2) consists of slow circular compression of soft tissues against underlying bone. The greatest pressure is applied as the hands move proximally, although contact is continuous. Small areas are usually treated using the fingertips alone. Kneading promotes the flow of tissue fluid and causes reflex vasodilation and marked **hyperaemia**. This reduces swelling, decreases muscle spasm and can stretch tissues shortened by injury.

> **hyperaemia**
> *an excessive amount of blood in the vessels supplying an organ or body part*

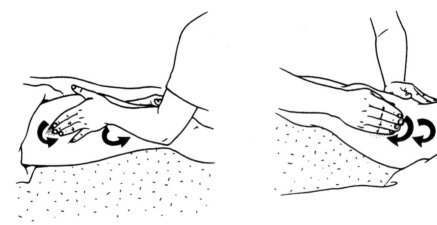

Figure 6.2 *Kneading*

Petrissage

Petrissage is particularly useful for stretching contracted or adherent fibrous tissue and will relieve muscle spasm. Acting more deeply than kneading, petrissage also promotes the flow of body fluids and can resolve long-standing swelling. Skin rolling is a forceful technique that can be applied only to fleshy regions of the body. A fold of skin, subcutaneous tissue and muscle is squeezed, lifted and rolled against the underlying tissues in a continuous circular motion. With each cycle, the hands progress on to adjacent tissue, taking care not to drag uncomfortably on the skin.

Two variants of the original technique have a more localised application and allow treatment of injuries in delicate soft tissue lying over superficial bone, such as an anterior tibial muscle strain. These are wringing and picking up. Wringing evolved from simple rolling petrissage; superficial tissues are grasped in both hands and twisted in opposite directions (Figure 6.3). Picking up involves lifting and stretching soft tissues away from underlying tissues (Figure 6.4).

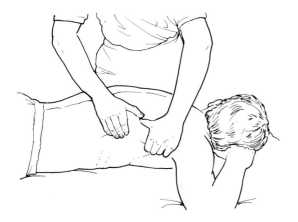
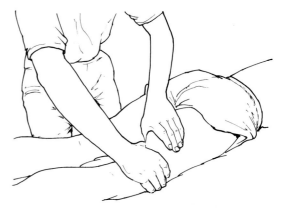
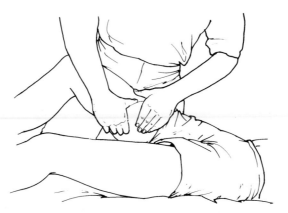

Figure **6.3** *Wringing*

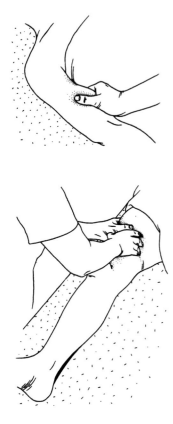

Figure 6.4   *Picking up*

Frictions

Frictions involves accurately delivering penetrating pressure through the fingertips or thumb. The movement is mainly circular or transverse relative to the alignment of the underlying structures with minimal lateral movement. Frictions are aimed directly at the site of damage (Figure 6.5). Tendons and ligaments are treated under slight tension, while muscles are best manipulated in a relaxed position, avoiding excessive damage to the muscle cells. The firm pressure needed for frictions is transmitted through the index finger, which is reinforced by the middle finger. Larger areas are treated using the index, middle and ring fingers of one hand supported by those of the other.

Friction massage begins with initial gentle transverse movements that gradually bear more deeply into the tissue and continue for 5–15 minutes. Frictions do not attempt to soothe, but cause mild tissue destruction, a marked local hyperaemia and an inflammatory reaction.

Frictions are very useful in sports therapy, especially for the treatment of adherent or contracted connective tissue – contracted tissue often significantly reduces athletic performance. The localised stretching and degradation of collagen caused by frictions can restore fibres to a more normal alignment during the remodelling phase of healing. Function often improves greatly, provided that healing is accompanied by correct joint positioning and gentle exercise.

This massage technique will also temporarily reduce pain by activating the 'pain gate' mechanism.

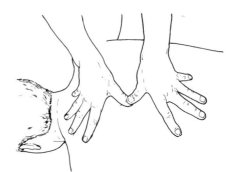

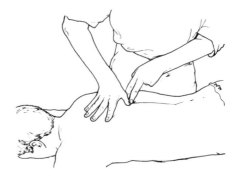

Figure 6.5   *Frictions*

Tapotement

Tapotement is the name given to percussive massage techniques. The purpose of these vigorous applications, which are often misunderstood, is to vibrate tissues, to trigger cutaneous reflexes and cause vasodilation. Thus muscle tone increases and retained interstitial fluid resulting from injury and inflammation is dispersed, swelling reduces and healing is accelerated.

There are several tapotement techniques, the simplest being 'cupping'. In this, the therapist cups his or her hands and strikes the patient's skin smartly with the concave air cushion next to the skin. This reduces the stinging sensation of the slap and disperses the shock more evenly through the tissues. Modifications of this basic technique, which have the same therapeutic effects, include

- hacking along the long axis of tissue using the ulnar border of the hand
- beating the skin with loosely flexed fingers
- pounding with tightly closed fists.

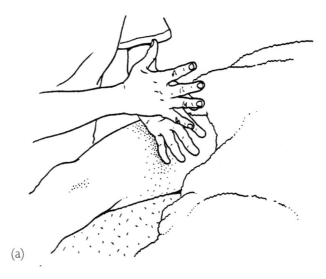

(a)

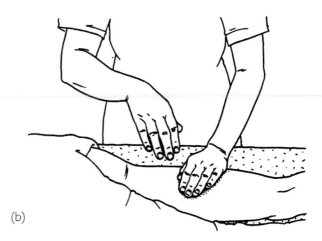

(b)

Figure 6.6 *Hacking (a) and cupping (b)*

Vibrations and shaking

These types of massage produce coarser and more energetic vibration of the tissue. Vibrations are delivered by trembling both hands firmly in contact with the skin. This method compresses swollen tissue and can reduce oedema, lessening the risk of infection spreading within natural channels in the body. Vibrations are also used by physiotherapists to disperse mucus from the smaller elements of the respiratory tree and to improve respiratory function.

Shaking is an even more vigorous treatment, in which the muscle of the chest wall is grasped and shaken forcefully.

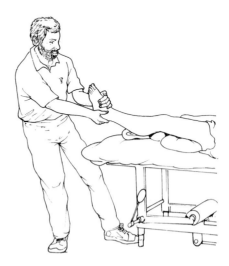

Figure 6.7   *Gentle shaking/rocking and vibrating*

PROGRESS CHECK
- What are the differences between pre-event massage and post-event massage?

Techniques using equipment

Devices increasing pressure

Rollers are the least sophisticated example of a family of devices that compress tissue. Massage using hand-held rollers was widespread about 1880. It is once again very popular in fitness centres. Rollers are available from most chemists or health shops. However, there is little evidence that this technique does more than soothe, an effect likely to depend more upon the skill of the masseur than upon the equipment itself.

Hydromassage

Rhythmically alternating external pressure, applied using warm flowing water, is the basis for many traditional hydrotherapy massage treatments. Hydrotherapy treatments include:

- undercurrent massage – application of a powerful underwater jet to the skin

- needle showers – fine but forceful jets of water are directed at a standing patient
- the whirlpool bath, or jacuzzi.

Hydromassage is often available in fitness clinics and should play an important role in sports therapy and sports rehabilitation. Hydromassage can cause deep relaxation, soften and debride scarred or hardened skin, and induce general vasodilation that accelerates healing of superficial tissues.

External compression

Pneumatic external compression, applied using an air-filled cuff or sleeve, has a history of successfully treating swollen limbs. Modern systems such as the 'Flowtron' (Huntleigh Technology, Luton) use an air compressor to rhythmically inflate and deflate a plastic sleeve wrapped around the limb. Pulsed pressure changes, within predetermined limits, alternately empty superficial veins and lymph channels into deep circulation, and then allow refilling. Valves within the deep vessels ensure unilateral flow.

Percussors

Percussors (one is shown in Figure 6.8) mimic the manual technique of tapotement. Their use is limited; they are perhaps most useful for the patient to use at home.

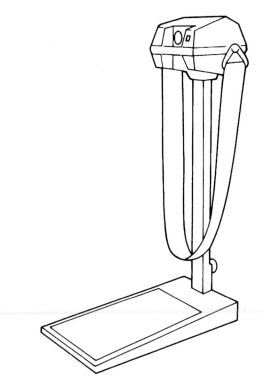

Figure 6.8 *Percussor*

Gyrators

A good gyrator will mimic the effects of manual body massage, although it is less effective. The principal advantage of this equipment that it produces a good massage in less time than a manual technique, something that you need to consider when you are out in the world working for yourself.

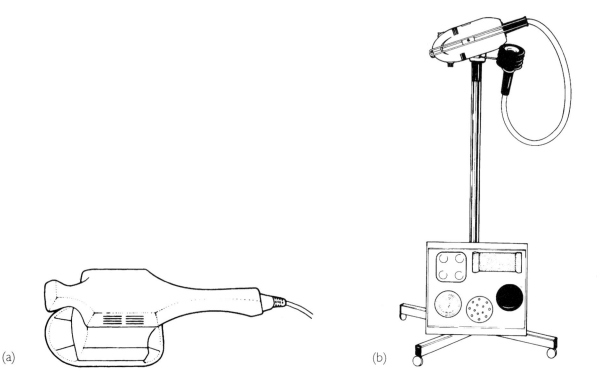

(a)

(b)

Figure 6.9 *A hand-held and pedestal gyrator*

PROGRESS CHECK
- Explain the meaning of the words palpation, effleurage, kneading, friction.
- What are the therapeutic effects of massage?
- What are the main contraindications to massage?
- How would you use hydromassage?

Heat and electrical therapies

The sports therapist is confronted with a bewildering array of commercial electrotherapy hardware that differs tremendously in effect, performance and price. Equipment is often marketed as a cure-all and may be backed by dubious endorsements and suspect research. You should be aware of the exact physiological effects to look for from the machine and should be familiar with the relevant research concerning these effects.

Non-heating therapies

Non-heating electrotherapeutic modalities include:

- interferential currents

- galvanic stimulation
- pulsed electromagnetic energy
- TENS
- low-dose pulsed ultrasound.

In general, all of these devices give some measure of pain relief, reduce muscle spasm, help to control the inflammatory process, help to reduce swelling and in some way enhance the healing process. For precise descriptions of the devices and their physiological responses you should look at the appropriate electrotherapy textbooks.

Heat therapy

A heating effect can be produced from many sources:

- infrared
- ultraviolet radiation
- hot water bottles
- massage
- showers
- baths.

All are methods of heating external tissues.

Short-wave and microwave diathermy, and continuous ultrasound, emit energy to create heat within the deeper tissues of the body, such as the muscles, tendons and ligaments. Dosages and administration of these complex devices must be left in the hands of the specially trained sports therapist.

The important therapeutic effects resulting from heat application are:

- *Pain relief*. A mild degree of heating relieves pain, presumably as a result of a sedative effect on the sensory nerves. It is most likely that this effect works through a mechanism similar to that of application of ice and TENS.
- *Relaxation of muscle spasm*. By relieving pain, associated muscle spasm and tension are also relieved. Muscles relax most readily when the tissues are warm.
- *Increased extensibility*. Heating the tissues increases muscle and ligament extensibility, which enhances easier stretching and facilitates muscle contractility.
- *Increased blood supply and metabolism*. The application of heat dilates the capillaries and arterioles in the immediate area, thus increasing the flow of blood. The supply of oxygen and foodstuffs to the area therefore increases and waste products are removed more rapidly. This increase in metabolism is greatest in the region where most heat is produced, resulting in an increase in the speed of the healing process.

However, it has been shown that the heat in a muscle during work or exercise is 10–20 times greater than the heat produced in a resting muscle. Exercise after injury is therefore an important means of accelerating metabolism – and in this regard is more efficient than applied heat. It is recommended that heat should be applied mainly for its analgesic effect and the relaxation of muscle spasm.

Ultrasound

Ultrasound is a form of deep heat and massage treatment in which high-frequency sound energy is produced by passing an alternating current through a quartz or quartz substitute crystal. The therapist either applies a coupling medium in the form of a gel to the injured part or treats the injured area in water.

Ultrasound energy passes through the skin and causes the body tissue to vibrate at its own frequency. This minute vibration acts like a micromassage, the depth of penetration depending on the frequency of the sound. One million cycles per second (1 MHz), for example, will penetrate more deeply than 3 MHz.

The ultrasound beam can be produced continuously or can be pulsed. The continuous beam produces a considerable amount of heat in the tissues. The pulsed beam produces little heat but still has the micromassaging effect. Generally the pulsed beam is used near bony surfaces to avoid possible damage to tissue through over-heating.

GOOD PRACTICE ▷ *Ultrasound is extremely dangerous if used inappropriately. For that reason any therapist must attend an approved course of study before using ultrasound.*

Regaining the components of fitness in the injured structure

After the acute (or immediate) reaction to injury has been controlled, rehabilitative exercises should be commenced.

Prolonged rest and immobilisation can delay early recovery (see Chapter 3). Because the resultant scar tissue is of poor quality, it is essential to begin appropriate exercises and activity to remodel and strengthen the new collagenous fibres. The implications for the athlete are considerable if this fact is not recognised.

The specific aims for rehabilitation at this stage are to regain flexibility, strength, endurance, power, co-ordination and skills leading to normal function of the injured structure.

Flexibility

It is important to regain flexibility, not only of the damaged structures but also of the muscles and ligaments around the damaged area. The best way permanently to lengthen and regain flexibility of connective tissue without compromising structural integrity is to use prolonged, low-intensity stretching at elevated tissue temperatures, and to cool the tissue before releasing the tension.

When the tissue is stretched, it may exhibit elastic or plastic properties, or a combination of both. Elastic stretch is a spring-like behaviour where the effect of the stretch is temporary or recoverable. In plastic stretch the tissue retains its new shape after the elongating stress is released. This permanent elongation is the desired result when dealing with scar tissue.

Temperature has a significant influence on the mechanical behaviour of tissues under tensile stress. Heating increases extensibility – recent studies have demonstrated that more plastic deformation will occur at about 44°C than at lower temperatures. Cooling the tissues before releasing the tension apparently allows the collagenous microstructure to restabilise towards its new stretched length.

Slow static stretching should be the technique of choice, as these procedures will override the protective stretch reflex and allow the muscle and any other damaged structures to increase in length.

A contract–relax technique is used with best effect. The muscle to be stretched (or the muscle controlling the joint or structure to be stretched) is resisted strongly in the opposite direction for 10 seconds. The patient is allowed 20 seconds for recovery and the process is repeated twice. To increase the chance of permanent plastic effects occurring, ice should then be applied for about 20 minutes with the structure in a sustained stretch.

Strength

Scar tissue is *never* as strong as the tissue it replaces. For rehabilitative purposes, strength should be considered in three categories:

- *Strength* – the maximum force that can be exerted in a single all-out effort. A weight lifter aims for this type of strength.
- *Power* – explosive action or the ability of a muscle to exert force with speed. High jumpers, boxers and shot-putters need to develop power.
- *Muscular endurance* – the ability of a muscle to contract repeatedly or to sustain a contraction against resistance. Long-distance runners, rowers, mountain climbers and cross-country skiers will need to develop this type of muscular fitness.

Depending on the particular sport and the individual's specific needs, the rehabilitation programme should be aimed at overloading one or more of these parameters.

To compensate for the lack of strength in the scar tissue, it is important for the athlete to participate in an intensive, well-planned strengthening programme. If the injury has occurred in a musculotendinous unit (such as a hamstring muscle), the patient must undergo a retraining programme to develop strength, power and endurance of the unit (depending on the sport played). For an injured joint, the athlete must strengthen the muscles controlling the joint as the joint tissues will strengthen as the muscular workload increases.

Where movement is restricted at any stage of rehabilitation (because of pain, swelling, spasm or plaster), isometric contractions serve the purpose until a progressive resistance programme of isotonic or isokinetic contractions can be instituted. An isometric exercise is one in which no joint movement occurs and the contraction is against a fixed resistance – for example the other hand, a doorway or wall. Each contraction should be applied with minimal pressure for a minimum of six seconds.

An isotonic exercise is one where there is a change in muscle length as a resistance is moved through a range of movement (for example a barbell, weight, boot or brick).

Isokinetics is a method of exercise at controlled speed and accommodating resistance. The muscle is made to work at its maximum capacity throughout its whole range of movement. It incorporates the factors of work, power, force and endurance through both isotonic and isometric exercises. The only drawback with this form of exercise is that it requires expensive specialised equipment.

It is clear, both from clinical observation and from experimental evidence, that a tissue is only as strong as the function placed on it. So, if you consider that a chain is only as strong as its weakest link, and the weak link is obviously the healing scar tissue, it is essential to design and implement a specific and general retraining programme.

This subject is covered further in Chapter 7.

Co-ordination

When soft tissue is injured, nerve endings and nerve pathways are inevitably damaged. When a joint capsule is damaged, a certain amount of **reflex arc** is lost. This leads to a lack of motor co-ordination, a tendency for joints to give way and for slowed reflexes when performing specific or general movements. It is therefore important to include co-ordination exercises in the rehabilitation programme. For instance, a cricketer with a damaged shoulder may need to undergo a programme incorporating the myotatic reflex for bowling. (When a muscle is stretched out fully, it initiates the myotatic reflex, which produces a stronger and faster contraction.) Similarly, a footballer with an ankle injury will need to regain motor co-ordination and **proprioception**. For players this mainly means balance and sense of joint position.

> **reflex arc**
> *the sequence of nerves involved in a reflex action*
>
> **proprioception**
> *the sum response to a great many different 'stimuli' sent to the brain or spinal cord by nerve endings in muscles and joints*

Regaining functional activity

As stated at the beginning of this chapter, rehabilitation must begin immediately after injury and continue until the patient is ready to return to their sport. Athletes must be restored to full competitive fitness at the earliest possible moment. It is important to recognise that an athlete has a much higher level of cardiovascular fitness (fitness of the heart and lungs) than an untrained individual. Athletes must, therefore, appreciate the urgency of dynamic early therapy to maintain this fitness. The importance of the 'treat and train' attitude has been effectively shown in studies of bed rest and training. When untrained subjects were rested for a 20-day period, it took them only 10 days to regain maximal oxygen intake (which is a measure of their cardiovascular fitness), but it took trained athletes up to 40 days to regain their previous fitness level.

Never let an athlete be idle because of injury. The rest of the body should still be made to work strongly – by swimming, running, punching, weight training or whatever they are capable of doing. Furthermore, they must begin to retrain for their sport as soon as possible while they are still receiving treatment for their specific injury. An athlete with a hamstring injury should start jogging (within limits of pain) as soon as possible; a tennis player with a 'tennis elbow' should start to play tennis at pain-free levels while the elbow condition is still being treated.

The point is that the damaged area must be retrained specifically through all the skills of the proposed sport so it can functionally adapt to the stresses of that sport.

All of these factors reinforce the need for the institution of an early, active, positively directed rehabilitation programme based on the need of the individual athlete.

PROGRESS CHECK

- What are the specific aims of the rehabilitation stage?
- Explain flexibility.
- Explain strength.
- Explain co-ordination.
- How do you know when your patient has returned to functional fitness?

KEY TERMS

You need to know what these words mean. Go back through the chapter or check the glossary to find out.

Rehabilitation	Spasm	Strength
Functional	Massage	Co-ordination
Pain	Acute	
Cryotherapy	Flexibility	

7 Fitness testing, training and avoidance of injury

After working through this chapter you will be able to:

➤ demonstrate an understanding of the principles of fitness testing
➤ use each piece of equipment
➤ devise an appropriate testing programme for injury
➤ advise on endurance, strength and speed
➤ design and implement appropriate training programmes for avoiding further injury.

Athletic performance today draws nearer and nearer to physiological limits and maximal human performance. Therefore, there is a fine line between injury-free performance and overstressing of the human body. Injury is the result of stress placed upon an organism which disrupts its structure and function and results in the pathological process of repair.

Classification of injury

Injuries can involve many factors. It is necessary to consider details such as physical fitness of the athlete, proficiency at their sport, psychological state and nutritional state. To gain a clear appreciation of the manner in which injury develops and to illustrate the complexity of sports injury, a classification of sports injury by causative factors given in Table 7.1.

Injuries will always occur when people are involved in sport and recreation, although steps can be taken to reduce the frequency and severity of injury. In industry the prevention of injury in the workplace is far more cost effective than treating the injury after it occurs – and the same applies to the sports arena. Surgery, hospitalisation and time off work for healing and rehabilitation place enormous financial burdens on the community.

Many factors can contribute to the development of an injury, as illustrated in Table 7.1. The athlete has direct control over many of these factors. Athletes should ensure that they:

• are fit enough to participate in the sport
• use effective warm-up and warm-down procedures
• wear appropriate clothing and protective devices
• do not infringe laws of the game to place themselves, or other participants, in danger.

Other factors are not under the control of the athletes but are within the province of sports coaches, administrators and umpires. Such areas include the imparting of the specific skills and techniques of sports, providing and maintaining correct, safe, hygienic facilities for sport, and ensuring the sport is played according to the appropriate rules and in the right spirit of competition.

Table 7.1 *Classification of injury in sport*

Consequential injury (due to sports participation)

PRIMARY

Extrinsic
1 Human – body contact sports (e.g. footballer's 'corked thigh' caused by an opponent's knee)
2 Implemental – caused by racquets, bats, balls and other implements necessary to carry out games
   a Instantaneous – due to immediate direct violence (e.g. blow received from a hockey stick)
   b Overuse – repeated stress of manipulating a sporting appliance (e.g. blisters on a rower's hands)
3 Vehicular (e.g. motorcyclist's crash)
4 Environmental – situations such as poor playing surface, bad lighting, faulty or damages implements, extreme weather conditions

Intrinsic (stress developed inside the body)
1 Instantaneous – e.g. a sprinter's pulled hamstring
2 Overuse
   a Acute – occurring in one incidence of sports participation (e.g. Achilles tendon strain)
   b Chronic – developing over a period (e.g. Achilles tendonitis)

SECONDARY

This injury occurs as a result of earlier injury which has been poorly treated or poorly diagnosed
1 Early – developing soon after the primary injury (e.g. quadriceps extensor mechanism malfunction)
2 Late – developing years after the injury (e.g. degenerative joint disease in an unstable joint)

Non-consequential injury
Injury and other conditions not directly caused by sport but which may interfere with participation in sport

---

Source: J.G.P. Williams, *Injury in Sport*, published by Wolfe Medical Publications, 1980.

PROGRESS CHECK

- What are the main factors that cause sports injury?
- What are the principal preventive measures for minimising injury in sport?

Prevention of injury

Preventive measures for minimising injury in sport can be grouped under six headings:

- pre-season medical examination
- fitness and training
- the warm-up
- athletic skill and coaching proficiency
- protective equipment
- miscellaneous factors.

The pre-season medical

A thorough medical examination should be undertaken and recorded at the beginning of every season. The purpose of the examination is to:

1 determine if there is any defect or condition that could place the athlete at risk or increase the chance of injury

2 bring to the attention of the therapist/athlete any weakness or imbalances, so that these problems can be corrected.

The examination could be carried out by a doctor but the sports therapist should also have access to the information from this examination. If there are minor problems, resolve them before they become major.

Fitness and training

Inadequate fitness or conditioning is a major contributor to sporting injuries. Lack of strength, power, endurance, flexibility or co-ordination at a vital moment may easily lead to breakdown of the body's tissues. The determined athlete's will to win will soon reveal a weak link resulting from a poorly designed training programme.

The purpose of training is to expose the body to repeated stresses of varying intensities and durations so that it will adapt to these stresses. Training science determines the demands on an athlete so that he or she will improve, and so that the stress will not become so severe as to prevent the body from being able to adapt, with eventual injury occurring. There are certain principles it is necessary to grasp.

REMEMBER

Fitness is a process of progressively adapting the body throughout training to withstand the rigours of competition.

PROGRESS CHECK

- What is fitness?
- Why is it important for a sports therapist to assess an athlete before their sporting season?

Principles of training

The main principles of fitness training are:

- progressive overload
- specificity

- relaxation
- routine.

Progressive overload

The training programme *must* be increased progressively so that the body is gradually challenged and placed under additional stress. Careful planning is important, as steadily augmented practice sessions should eliminate calf and shin soreness and most of the minor muscle strains associated with overtraining. A progressive overload is implemented by increasing one or more of the following:

- the amount of resistance
- the repetition of sets
- the intensity (rate) of the exercise
- the duration of the work or exercise.

Specificity

Specificity is the overriding consideration in planning and implementing all training programmes. The type of programme must apply appropriate stress to the specific components of an athlete's body to enable him or her to undertake a specific task. Therefore the type of sport and the position in the team for which the individual is training must be considered. For example, in rugby, as well as a general conditioning programme the outside backs should concentrate on strengthening their calves, quadriceps and hamstrings. The front row forwards should concentrate on strengthening their backs, shoulder and neck muscles for scrummaging. The design of a programme for a 100-m sprinter would be vastly different from that for a marathon runner.

ACTIVITY

Choose six sports. Using your knowledge of the muscles of the body and Figure 7.1 identify the muscles used in each sport.

Relaxation

The body needs time to recover from hard exercise. Adequate rest is necessary to allow recuperation and repair of any damage suffered during a hard training session. Training should allow for 'hard–easy' days. Heavy sessions should occur only three to four times a week with light workouts in between. Lack of adequate rest or sleep may result in:

- physiological staleness, characterised by a decreased ability to perform and muscle fatigue, or
- psychological staleness, characterised by a loss of interest in training or competing.

Routine

Fitness training is a continual process and it must be done regularly, throughout the year. As well as an overall season plan, there should be both weekly and daily plans. It is the responsibility of the coach or the sports therapist to monitor an athlete's performance, making sure they are not overworked, that they are getting adequate sleep and that they are eating a balanced diet.

Activity Chart

Sport: _____

Position: _____

Body Area	Muscles Used
Upper Body	
Arm	
Trunk (including back)	
Leg	

Figure 7.1 *Activity chart*

Components of fitness

Physical fitness can be broken down into a number of components:

- cardiovascular endurance
- muscular strength, power and endurance
- flexibility.

It is important to understand how each of these components adapts to the training.

Cardiovascular endurance

The ability of an athlete to sustain repeated muscular effort requires the respiratory system, the heart and the blood vessels to deliver fuel and oxygen to the muscles at a rate fast enough to prolong the time before fatigue sets in. Fatigue will leave the athlete vulnerable to injury.

Aerobic training

Aerobic training is the term used to describe the development of cardiovascular endurance, and certain variables must be considered to gain necessary adaptations.

The intensity of the programme can be easily determined by the response of the heart rate to exercises. The maximum heart rate of an individual can be calculated by the simple formula:

220 minus the age of the athlete

Therefore the maximum heart rate for a 20-year-old adult would be about 200 beats per minute. To increase cardiovascular endurance an athlete should work at 80% of their maximal heart rate. For a 20-year-old athlete this would be 160 beats per minute.

ACTIVITY

Calculate your own maximal heart rate.

REMEMBER

As cardiovascular endurance improves, the heart rate drops.

A workout session of a least 30 minutes maintaining the target heart rate is the minimum necessary to produce significant changes.

A minimum of three sessions of aerobic activity should be followed per week. The cardiovascular system will adapt to exercise in various ways:

- the heart, which is specialised muscle, will increase in thickness and therefore become a more efficient pump, producing an increased stroke volume and cardiac output, increasing blood supply to the muscles
- there will be an increased ability to extract oxygen from the air breathed into the lungs
- the blood vessels, especially the smaller ones (capillaries), will show a decrease in resistance to blood flow.

Anaerobic conditioning

The anaerobic system is the local muscle energy system that is used in the absence of oxygen. It is used in explosive body movements which occur before oxygen can be delivered to the muscle. To train this system, rapid explosive movements of short duration are necessary – for example, short sprints. Therefore, a training programme should strike a balance between long-distance endurance work (aerobic) and short, intensive fast work (anaerobic).

PROGRESS CHECK

What are the three components of fitness?

Muscular parameters

A muscle can develop strength, power and endurance.

Strength

A muscle's strength is defined as the maximum force it can develop against a resistance, and is proportional to the cross-sectional area of the muscle. When a muscle is subjected to high-intensity demands, it will respond by increasing in size and strength. Best strength gains are achieved by a regime of high resistance and low repetition. When devising a strength programme, select:

- the type of resistance
- the amount of resistance to be applied
- the number of repetitions per set
- the number of sets per workout
- the number of workouts per week.

Table 7.2 *Resistance-using strength training*

Types of resistance	Type of movement	Device used
Isometric	No movement, contraction against a fixed resistance; each contraction held for 6 seconds	Any immovable object
Isotonic	These are contractions where the muscle changes length against a resistance	Free weights, wall pulleys (e.g. Universal, Nautilus)
Isokinetic	These contractions require a specialised device which allows an accommodating resistance; that is, the resistance adapts throughout the range of motion	Cybex, Orthotron, Hydragym

Power

Power is the rate of doing work. It is the ability of the muscle to exert a force at accelerated speed, therefore explosive contractions are required. Power is best developed using isokinetic machines.

Endurance

This is the ability of the muscle to contract repeatedly. Athletes need to use a high percentage of that strength over a period of time through repeated muscular contractions. Best endurance gains are achieved with moderate resistance and high repetitions. To set an endurance programme:

- select a low resistance
- increase the rate of work
- increase the number of repetitions and sets.

Flexibility

Lack of flexibility is a common cause of injury to muscles and joints. Increasing flexibility through controlled stretching may decrease the incidence of musculotendinous injury, minimise and alleviate muscle soreness, and contribute to improved athletic performance. A muscle must achieve full stretch before it can attain its full power. Similarly, a ligament or a tendon must be long enough to allow a joint to move fully through its normal range of motion and achieve efficient function. Therefore, to prevent injury, athletes should carry out regular stretching exercises to ensure flexibility and full range of motion of joints and muscles.

The stretching technique and the methods used to incorporate stretching exercises in an overall fitness plan are crucial to the development of a safe, effective programme. Poor technique and improper stretching may actually cause musculotendinous injury. Increases in flexibility should be attained by slow, gentle, static stretches. Static stretching allows the muscle's protective reflex, the stretch reflex, to be overcome. The muscle is then relaxed and can be stretched further, safely. The athlete should hold the position of stretch for 10–15 seconds. There should be no excess straining, bouncing or pain. As flexibility improves, the duration of the stretch can be increased to 30 seconds or more. This is the safest and most effective method of increasing flexibility.

Ballistic stretches (for example, high kicks), bouncing in the stretched position, or rapid movements during a stretch are all counter-productive. This is because a muscle will contract reflexively when it is suddenly stretched (this is the stretch reflex). Therefore, any fast bouncing stretch will be against a contracted muscle – which may injure the muscle tissue if it is forced or will not produce any significant stretching of the muscle.

Planning a stretching programme

It is important to realise that increasing flexibility is a gradual progression – it will take many weeks before any benefit can be seen. Athletes should be encouraged to develop a year-round programme. Stretching at the beginning of a season will have only minimal benefits.

Stretching should always be preceded by a mild aerobic warm-up (a mild, repetitive activity such as jogging or cycling). This warms the muscles and increases their extensibility, which helps to protect them against injury and allows greater gains in flexibility. Stretching and an effective warm-up should precede all physical activity. Further stretching can also be undertaken during a workout routine when the muscles are warm and extensible. Stretching after a heavy workout is an excellent way to relax muscles and minimise muscle soreness.

Muscle groups should be alternated throughout the stretching routine. If, for example, the routine starts with a quadriceps stretch, the next exercise should be for some other group, such as the calf muscles. Spacing the various exercises will avoid excessive force on any one muscle group. Suitable stretches are shown in Figure 7.2.

REMEMBER

Poor technique and improper stretching can actually cause injury.

REMEMBER

Slow, static stretching will override the stretch reflex and allow the muscle to increase in length.

Table 7.3 *Summary of stretching*

Precede stretching with a mild aerobic warm-up

Use the static stretching technique

The stretching position should be assumed slowly and gently until tightness is experienced. This position is held for 15 or more seconds. There should be no pain, and no bouncing or jerky movements

Exercise the various muscle groups alternately

Stretch before, after and (if possible) during the exercise sessions. If there is time for only one routine, stretching before the activity is the most important

Plan a year-round stretching routine

Partner stretching – the contract–relax method

Many people have some muscle groups that are particularly tight and find difficulty in relaxing them to gain a significant stretch. Stretching with a partner will aid these people.

- The athlete moves the limb in the direction to be stretched until a feeling of tension is experienced, and holds it for 10 seconds.
- The limb is then forced against a resistance applied by the partner in the opposite direction to that being stretched. The partner provides an isometric resistance (no movement). The contraction is held for 6 seconds.
- The muscle is allowed to relax and is then moved by the partner – gently – in the direction to be stretched. This new stretch is held for 10 seconds.

The procedure is repeated four or five times. If it is done correctly relaxation of the muscle and an increase in flexibility will be noted.

PERFORMANCE CHECK

- How can added flexibility assist in prevention of injury?
- Explain progressive overload.
- Why is relaxation so important?

The warm-up

The warm-up is an integral part of injury prevention as it prepares the athlete's body and mind for competition. A warm-up should

1   Ensure complete flexibility of all joints and muscles
2   Ensure proper muscle contractility for sudden explosive action
3   Raise aerobic energy supply
4   Refresh skill patterns
5   Aid psychological preparation for sport.

Exercise increases body temperature, and flexibility increases as body temperature rises. An increase in muscle temperature enables enzyme systems to work more rapidly and improves the viscosity of tissues. This

Shoulders

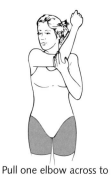

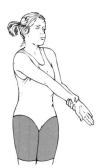

Pull one elbow across to the opposite shoulder

Pull one arm across the body, thumb towards the ground

Pectoral muscles

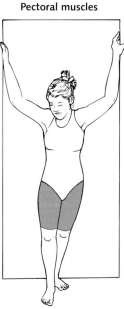

Stand in a doorway. Lean your body forward

Biceps

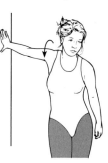

Hold onto a door at arm's length, thumb down. Turn your body away from that arm; let the shoulder roll in

Outer thigh

Place the leg to be stretched behind the other leg, keeping the first leg straight. Let the front knee relax as you rotate and bend away from the leg to be stretched

Latissimus dorsi

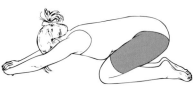

Raise your hands over your head and stretch forward as shown. Then, with hips in the air and hands on the floor, lean hips towards the side to be stretched. Feel the stretch from shoulder blade to armpit

Triceps

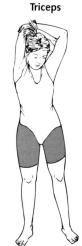

Place one hand behind your head. Pull the elbow behind your head with the opposite hand

Back extensors

Hip flexors

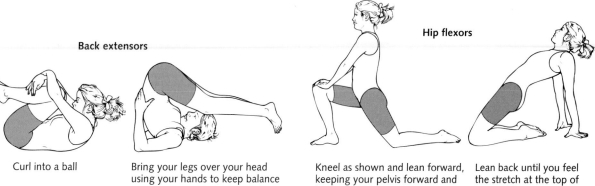

Curl into a ball

Bring your legs over your head using your hands to keep balance

Kneel as shown and lean forward, keeping your pelvis forward and back straight

Lean back until you feel the stretch at the top of your thigh

***Figure* 7.2**   *Stretching*

Calf muscles

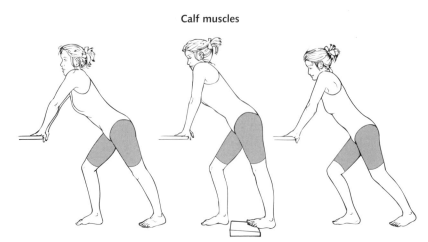

To stretch the gastrocnemius muscle, have feet and body pointing forwards and back straight. Lean forward; your heels must remain on the ground

A better stretch can be obtained by using an incline board

To stretch the soleus muscle, use the same position as for the gastrocnemius, then bend your knee to isolate the soleus

Wrist/forearm extensors

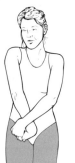

With elbow straight, pull on the back of your hand

Wrist/forearm flexors

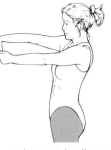

With a straight elbow, pull on the palm of your hand until you feel the stretch in your forearm

Buttock stretch

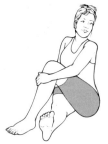

Keep both buttocks on the ground, with your back straight. Press against one knee as shown, while turning that leg away from the body

Hamstrings

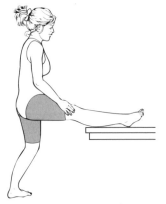

Standing up, place one leg on a bench. Bend the opposite knee to lock low back. With back straight, lean forwards

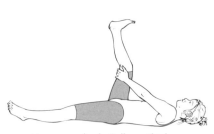

Lie on your back. Pull one thigh up with both hands, then straighten the knee

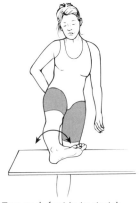

Turn each foot in to stretch the lateral hamstrings – out to stretch the medial hamstrings

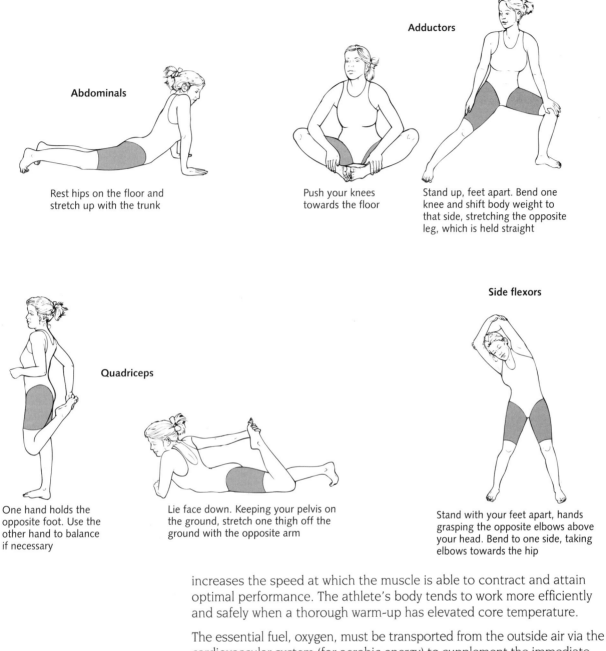

Abdominals

Rest hips on the floor and stretch up with the trunk

Adductors

Push your knees towards the floor

Stand up, feet apart. Bend one knee and shift body weight to that side, stretching the opposite leg, which is held straight

Quadriceps

One hand holds the opposite foot. Use the other hand to balance if necessary

Lie face down. Keeping your pelvis on the ground, stretch one thigh off the ground with the opposite arm

Side flexors

Stand with your feet apart, hands grasping the opposite elbows above your head. Bend to one side, taking elbows towards the hip

increases the speed at which the muscle is able to contract and attain optimal performance. The athlete's body tends to work more efficiently and safely when a thorough warm-up has elevated core temperature.

The essential fuel, oxygen, must be transported from the outside air via the cardiovascular system (for aerobic energy) to supplement the immediate source of energy contained in the muscles (the anaerobic energy). A slow, steady run will raise the maximum oxygen uptake, elevate the heart rate and reduce the resistance to blood flow, therefore attaining maximum efficiency of the aerobic energy supply system. If fast powerful sprinting work is done too early the athlete will use up their anaerobic energy supply before the aerobic supply can reach the muscle, causing the lactate level (waste products) in the blood to rise. This will lead to early fatigue.

Where possible, the warm-up session should reproduce the actual movements of the sport to be played. This will activate the neuromuscular pathways that are necessary to attain the specific skills of a sport, such as passing, throwing and kicking.

The intensity and duration of a warm-up should be governed by the type of event and the fitness of the athlete. As a general rule, trained athletes should warm up for approximately 20-30 minutes before competing. It is important for the athlete to understand the need to stay warm until the competition starts and to remain warm during the actual event. For instance, a rugby winger waiting for the ball to come his way must continually stretch and exercise to stay warm if he wants to avoid muscle or joint injury.

A *warm-up routine*

1   Slow steady jog for approximately 5 minutes. Slow jogging will raise the aerobic capacity and increase core temperature of the body

2   Stretching routine – approximately 10 minutes. This should stretch all major joints and muscles starting at the neck and systematically working down the body. Special attention must be placed on the muscles of the lower limbs and back, which are more susceptible to injury

3   Running – approximately 5 minutes. Progressive running drills over varying distances and increasing speeds should be given until the athlete has reached full pace over 75–100 m. Leg stretches should be interspersed with the running drills.

4   Skill – approximately 10 minutes. The activities and skills that the athlete will perform during the event should be practised during this period. For example, netball players should practise passing and goal shooting, sprinters their starts, footballers kicking and passing. It is also useful to run through the planned moves that the team will attempt during the course of the match.

5   Rest – a period of 10 minutes or so should be allowed for the athlete to relax before competition. Last-minute equipment and clothing checks should be carried out and the final psychological preparations made during this period

6   Warm-down – for 3–5 minutes after the event. This removes waste products (lactates) from the muscles and may help to reduce much of the post-match stiffness and soreness. Stretching will also help tired muscles to relax.

The role of the coach or sports therapist in teaching the correct techniques and skills of the sport to the athlete is an important factor in maintaining injury-free performance. For example:

- incorrect technique in a javelin throw can lead to elbow injury
- the fast bowler with an improper action may suffer low back pain
- an excessive 'whip kick' can cause pain in the breaststroker's knee.

PROGRESS CHECK   What is the purpose of the warm-up and what are its components?

Athletic skill and coaching proficiency

Many sports coaches and therapists are engaged because they used to play that particular sport. These people, although they are well intentioned, often lack the scientific knowledge concerning fitness training, skill development and prevention of injury.

Referees, coaches and therapists all have a responsibility to ensure that athletic endeavour is carried out within the rules and spirit of the game. Acts of premeditated violence, or intentional cheating risking injury to an opponent, must be eliminated from sport.

Protective equipment

A prime example of the use of protective equipment in sport is the equipment used in American football – no other sport uses such a vast array of protective pads, guards, facial protectors and strapping. Cricket is also becoming a gladiatorial game, due to the strength and power of the modern fast bowler. Consequently, in the last few years the variety of protective equipment used by batters to protect vulnerable parts of their body from damage by the impact of a cricket ball has increased (Figure 7.3).

Protective equipment used in sport must incorporate the following features in its design.

- Padding should be made of light materials, comfortable to wear and allowing adequate ventilation, particularly in a hot climate
- The device should not restrict movement or the normal function of the body – protective equipment should not hinder an athlete's ability to perform
- The protective device should be appropriate for the sport being played, and not breach the rules of the sport or be capable of being used as a weapon. However, in many sports there are no design specifications for protective equipment and poorly designed, inappropriate, devices can give a false sense of security
- The materials used should be capable of reducing the full force of impact over the body part to be protected.

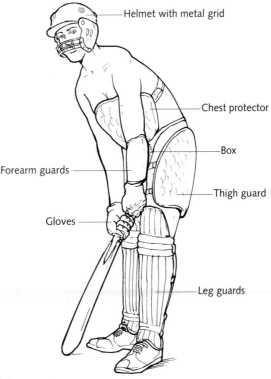

Figure 7.3   *Cricket protection*

Suitable protection:

- Mouthguards. These must be worn in all contact sports. Mouthguards are designed to protect the teeth and jaws against impact and have a role to play in reducing concussion.

- Bracing. The bracing of joints, particularly the knee, is becoming widespread.
- Taping. There is some evidence to suggest that the taping of ankles might help to prevent ankle joint injuries.

Miscellaneous factors

Diet

Appropriate food intake plays an essential role in injury prevention by supplying the necessary energy to guard against early fatigue. A well-balanced nutritious diet is needed to maintain health and fitness. Information and guidelines relating to diet can be found in Chapter 9.

Fluid replenishment

An adequate intake of water is essential before and during competition and training to prevent dehydration, cramping and heart stress. During heavy exercise, an athlete can lose up to 4–5 kg of body fluid. No matter how much a person drinks, they cannot keep up with such fluid losses during training and competition. Consequently, an athlete should drink 400–500 ml of fluid 10–15 minutes before competition and take in small amounts as often as possible during the event.

Hygiene

Athletes must be careful about their personal hygiene, for their own protection and that of their fellow athletes. This is especially important in team sports, particularly when travelling where infection and disease can easily spread to team mates. It is essential to clean and treat skin wounds, no matter how trivial, to prevent infection.

Fitness testing

To test someone's fitness successfully you need to:

- know their level of fitness before the injury
- know and understand the physical demands placed on the athlete in their sport
- understand that sport sufficiently to design appropriate tests.

Guidelines are given here for *general* fitness testing – but remember that each sport has specific demands over and above these.

Testing aerobic performance

Although the aerobic capacity can be measured properly only by using elaborate laboratory equipment, there are some relatively simple field tests that a therapist or coach can use which will give good comparative results. These tests produce only *relative* figures, and should be repeated at suitable intervals – for example weekly or monthly – for a pattern of improvement to show. The therapist or coach should be responsible for keeping the records.

The step test

This is easy to perform. All you need are:

- a step (50 cm for men, 45 cm for women and 38 cm for children)
- a timing clock or stop watch
- a metronome (visual ones are better than the electronic 'bleeping' types) – although this is not essential.

The most severe version of the test is 5 minutes of stepping at a rate of 30 steps per minute (metronome setting of 120, as each step has four beats). The procedure is to step the subjects for the appropriate period, making sure that they stand fully upright each time at the top of the step, then to rest them in a sitting position for 1 minute. The pulse rate is then measured for 30 seconds. Be sure to stop the metronome before you start counting – it is easy to get confused. So far you have two figures. First, the time in seconds (which will, of course, be 300 if the test was completed – if a subject cannot step for the full 5 minutes, simply note the overall time he or she completed). The second figure is the pulse count for 30 seconds, which will usually be between 40 and 65. Do *not* double this 30 second count: it goes into the formula as it is. Then you fit these two figures into a formula to give a simple 'fitness index' (FI):

$$FI = \frac{(\text{time in seconds}) \times 100}{(\text{pulse count for 30 seconds}) \times 5.5}$$

For example:

$$FI = \frac{300 \times 100}{42 \times 5.5} = 130$$

The higher the fitness index in this test the better. Very roughly, for the 5 minute test:

180 or above is superb

160–170 is excellent

140–159 is very good

120–139 is good

100–119 is creditable

80–99 is reasonable

It is simple to devise easier variants of the test; for example, with step rates of 20 or 25 and/or a shorter time of 4 minutes. Naturally, the scores cannot then be directly compared with those above. At the lower levels it is best for the therapist/coach to compile their own norms.

Pulse rate test
The simplest test of all in this category is to count and record the pulse rate first thing in the morning. However, this should only be taken as a broad guide, as individuals vary greatly. For example, a subject with a pulse rate in the 40s will usually be very fit in cardiorespiratory terms, but someone with a pulse rate of 70 is not necessarily unfit; some large strong trained hearts simply 'choose' to beat faster at rest than they otherwise could. As with all these fitness tests, it is the *pattern* they reveal which is the valid indicator or progress.

Speed training and testing drills

Anaerobic field testing

There is no field test for anaerobic muscle endurance comparable with, say, the step test for cardiorespiratory endurance. Therefore each sport tends to have its own particular tests. These take the form of a variety of movements, such as dips, squat jumps or star jumps, measured as the number completed in 30 or 60 seconds. If they are well related to the sport in question and backed by the experience of the therapist or coach, then such tests, repeated at intervals over reasonably long period, will give a good indication of improvement (or otherwise).

Running on the spot

Here is a typical example: partners face each other 1 m apart and run on the spot. They encourage each other to lift their knees high, exaggerate the arm movements, keep the shoulders square and look straight at their partner. Repeat in sets:

- half speed for 20–30 seconds, with 60 seconds recovery
- three-quarter speed for 20–30 seconds with 60 seconds recovery
- full speed for 10–15 seconds with 60 seconds recovery.

Speed endurance exercises

Exercises that can be used are shown in Figure 7.4. These exercises can be performed in sets with the recovery periods adjusted to suit the fitness level of the athlete.

Sprint training

- Sprint-assisted training – downhill running, towing and treadmill running all appear to contribute to increases in stride length and frequency.
- Sprint-resisted training – uphill running, clothing ballast and sand dune running all appear to increase the strength and aerobic and muscular endurance.
- Acceleration sprints – these gradually increase from a rolling start, through jogging, to striding out and eventually to maximum pace. This exercise is particularly useful for emphasising and maintaining the technical component of the sprinting action as speed increases.
- Hollow sprints
- Use brief sprints interrupted by a period of recovery in the form of light running or jogging. For example, accelerate for 30–50 m, jog 30–50 m, accelerate again for 30–50 m, then walk for 100–150 m as the recovery phase. This form of training is appropriate to games players as it offers a variation in speed and tempo within each sequence.
- Repetition sprints – this involves running fixed distances at constant speed (75–100% of maximum speed), with recovery periods of sufficient length to allow the athlete to maintain form and the required degree of quality.

Speed/power tests

There are a number of ways of measuring power, some of which use quite sophisticated laboratory equipment, but here are some examples of simple field tests which can be set up easily.

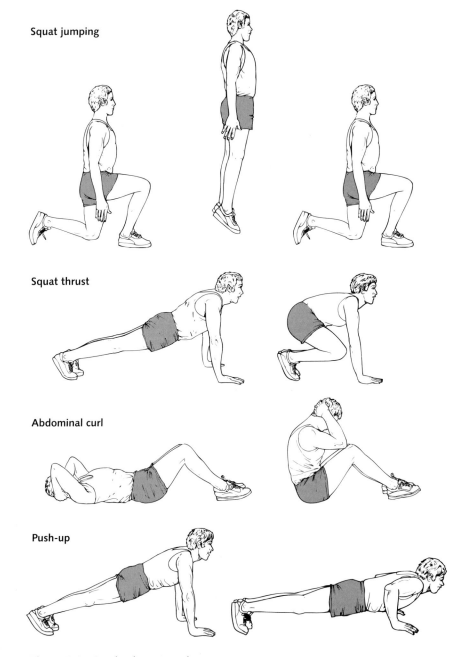

Figure 7.4 *Speed endurance exercises*

- *Vertical jump test* (Figure 7.5). Stand next to the wall, and reach as high as possible with one hand, noting the height. By bending and explosively extending the knees, jump vertically to touch the wall with the extended hand. Taking the best of three attempts, note the height reached by the top of the fingers and measure the distance between that and the point reached when standing.
- *Standing broad jump*. Stand with the toes just behind the line; swing the arms and spring forward from both feet. Taking the best of three attempts, measure from the line to the nearest heel mark.

- *Medicine ball throw.* Lie on the back, with arms extended above the head holding a medicine ball. By pulling forward with the arms only, and keeping the back flat to the floor, throw the ball over the feet as far as possible. Again taking the best of three attempts, measure the distance from the starting point of the medicine ball to the point where it lands.

- *Sprint tests.* You can easily devise short timed sprints on the athletics track or other suitable surface. Try standing-start tests over 20, 30, 40 or 50 metres. A useful variation is the flying start test: after a fixed run-in distance, say 20 m, the athlete is timed at full speed over the next 25 m.

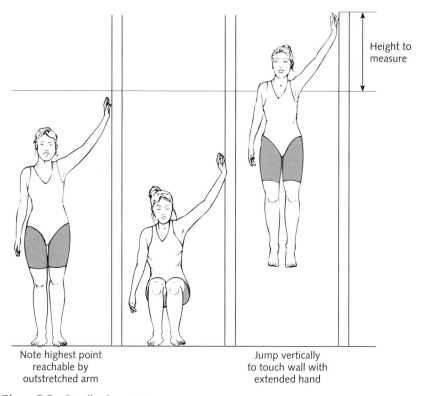

Height to measure

Note highest point reachable by outstretched arm

Jump vertically to touch wall with extended hand

Figure 7.5   *Standing jump test*

Development of strength

While relatively few sporting activities depend on pure strength alone, the performer who wishes to improve in any discipline will almost inevitably find that an increase in strength will be needed in certain areas. Muscular strength is generally built up by encouraging the muscle or group of muscles concerned to exert a force while contracting against a resistance. This contraction involves an increase in muscle tension. When this is repeated frequently, the muscle responds by accepting an increased flow of nutrients which in turn gives it the ability to deliver more power.

ACTIVITY

Before we look at strength exercises in detail, first refresh your memory about the different types of muscular contraction:

concentric is _____?

eccentric is _____?

isometric is _____?

isokinetic is _____?

Principles of strength training

Let's now look at the chief principles which form the basis for planning strength training programmes.

Overload

Muscular strength is most effectively developed when the muscle or group of muscles is overloaded by contracting against resistances exceeding those normally encountered. This forces the muscle to contract maximally (or near-maximally), which stimulates the physiological adaptations leading to increased muscular strength.

Progressive resistance

Muscles gain in strength as a result of training, which means that the initial overload will no longer provide the right degree of resistance to match progressive gains in strength. The loads against which a muscle is exercising must therefore be increased periodically and progressively throughout the course of a strength-training programme,

Specificity

You must appreciate that the response to training is specific, and the strength programmes that you devise must reflect the specific requirements of the sport. This is not simply a matter of exercising the muscle groups involved in particular movements – for best results the exercises must be directly related to the pattern and execution of those movements.

Reversibility

Much of the adaptation achieved from training is reversible, so the programme should be not only progressive but also continuous, avoiding prolonged periods of absence from training. It is common in training programmes for the performance to deteriorate during the early stages. This is because the body requires time to adapt to the overload being applied. Use your skills as a therapist or coach to prevent your performer from becoming disheartened at this critical early stage.

The strength training programme

Preliminary considerations

Before you devise the sequence of exercises in a strength training programme, you must consider the following factors.

- What is the nature and type of strength required? Everyone should start by developing general strength, but then the subsequent programme should be tailored to the individual and their sport.
- Which muscle/muscle groups are to be used? A careful analysis of the muscles involved is needed, followed by the selection of a suitable set of exercises.
- What is the range and variety of strength training methods available? You need to understand the application and relative effectiveness of
  - body resistance exercises
  - free weights
  - multi-station units
  - isometric training
  - isokinetic training

    – plyometrics (explosive power training)
    – pulleys and springs.

- How will you record and monitor progress? The best way is to keep a written schedule of the programme, with provision for regular progress evaluations.

Safety

You should be familiar with the recommendations below:

- As with all other forms of training, it is essential to warm up before strength training. This should include flexibility work both before and after the session.
- Whatever exercise is used, the correct principles of lifting should be learned, including correct breathing (Figure 7.6).
- Sensible resistances (loading) should be used at first. It is dangerous to lift excessively heavy weights too soon. If the starting weight is kept low in the early stages, the technique will be mastered much more quickly.
- Be aware of, and avoid, exercises or faulty body positions which may damage vulnerable parts of the body such as the back and the knees.
- Make sure that the training area is suitable: there should be adequate space, with safe footing. The floor must be even, firm and non-slip.
- Any equipment used should be soundly constructed, regularly checked and properly maintained.
- Expert instruction and supervision must be sought when specialised equipment is to be used.

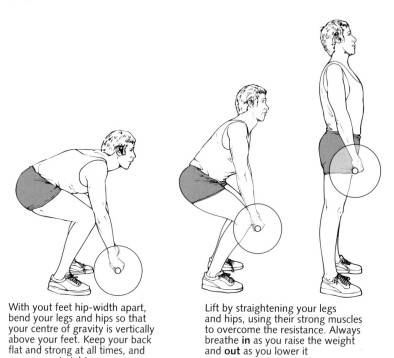

With yout feet hip-width apart, bend your legs and hips so that your centre of gravity is vertically above your feet. Keep your back flat and strong at all times, and your arms straight

Lift by straightening your legs and hips, using their strong muscles to overcome the resistance. Always breathe **in** as you raise the weight and **out** as you lower it

Figure 7.6   *The correct method of lifting is vital if you want to avoid back injury. It applies equally to lifting barbells and suitcases!*

Once you are satisfied that you have the correct knowledge and equipment, you can begin to think about the details of the programme:

Repetitions and sets

Repetitions (often shortened to 'reps') are the number of times an exercise is performed without stopping. A resistance is the load that the muscle (or group of muscles) is required to move.

An important concept to understand is the 'repetition maximum' (RM). A repetition maximum is defined as the maximum load a muscle or group of muscles can lift a given number of times before fatiguing. For example, if someone can do the bench press exercise ten times and no more before fatiguing, the weight used is the 10 RM load on that exercise for that person. The load (or resistance) used will depend on the type of strength to be developed. Exercises that involve high repetitions and low resistances will improve the endurance qualities of the muscle – low repetitions with high resistances develop pure strength.

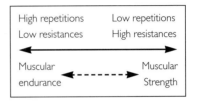

Figure 7.7 *Developing muscular endurance and strength*

A specific number of repetitions make up one set. For example, three sets of ten repetitions will be written as: 3 x 10.

It is not possible to state categorically the particular combinations of sets and RM load that will increase either muscular strength or muscular endurance most effectively – this depends on the individual and the specific requirements of the sport. However, significant strength gains can be achieved from programmes that consist of between one and six sets, with loads varying from 3 RM to 20 RM, so these figures can be used as a broad guide only. Most programmes consist of between one and three sets and loads of 5–10 RM.

Frequency and duration

It is generally agreed that two or three exercise sessions per week produce significant gains in strength. This should prevent excessive stress on an athlete by giving adequate recovery time between the sessions. Each session should normally last between 30 minutes and 1 hour, but this of course depends on the physical condition of the individual, the particular adaptations being sought, and the speed at which the exercise routines are carried out.

Speed

The optimum speed of a repetition will vary, depending on the muscle group being used and the specific requirements of the sport. You must appreciate that if the movement is speeded up the duration will shorten, and so reduce the strengthening effect of the exercise. Faster repetitions are likely to produce a more dynamic kind of strength, mainly through nerve adaptations, while slower movements tend to produce adaptations within the composition of the muscle.

Rest

Rest between repetitions should be minimal (less than 1 second). Rest intervals between sets should be 1.5–2 minutes, depending on the intensity of the session. Bearing the need for rest in mind, it is advisable to exercise the larger, more powerful, muscle groups before the smaller ones. This allows effective overload in the large muscles because the smaller groups fatigue more easily. So start working on the larger (leg and hip) muscles before moving to the smaller (arm) muscles. Sequences should not include successive exercises which use the same muscle groups. For example, working the upper legs and hips followed by the shoulders, back, lower leg, abdominals and finally the arms, would be a reasonable sequence, but this will obviously need to be varied according to the sport and the individual.

Maintaining strength levels

It is generally considered that one-third of the intensity of the original strength training programme is required to maintain the levels of strength achieved. Therefore if the original schedule for strength gain included three sessions per week, then continuing with one session per week should maintain the required level.

Types of strength programme

There is obviously considerable scope for variety in strength training programmes, but one well established approach is that devised by De Lorme and Watkins, who first developed the concept of the 'repetition maximum'. In their original schedule, each training session contained three sets of ten repetitions of each exercise, thus giving a total of 30 repetitions per muscle/group. The load is increased in each set:

Set 1:   10 reps at a load of half 10 RM
Set 2:   10 reps at a load of three-quarters 10 RM
Set 3:   10 reps at a load of 10 RM

From session to session the number of repetitions is increased while maintaining the same resistance load. The load is increased as soon as more than 10 repetitions are possible when performing set 3. The most effective part of this programme is the third set, which represents the greater resistance for the muscle group – although of course you cannot omit the first two sets.

A second well-proven programme uses the 'pyramid' approach. Again there is much possible variation, but the basic system requires that you first establish the maximum weight your subject can handle in a single lift (1 RM). You then devise a schedule based on increasing the load while decreasing the number of repetitions. For example:

Set 1:   8 repetitions at 50% of established maximum
Set 2:   4 repetitions at 75% of established maximum
Set 3:   1 repetition at 95% of the established maximum.

As with De Lorme and Watkins' programme, the load is increased as the subject improves. As soon as more than a single repetition is achieved in set 3, the load is raised to provide a new value for 1 RM.

Methods of strength training

Body resistance exercises

The most readily available form of resistance (load) is the body itself. Although there has been a considerable increase in weight-training facilities, equipment may not be available or convenient for your athlete or group of athletes to use. Using the body as the load allows some strength work during or after any other form of training or practice. As little special equipment is needed, it may take place almost anywhere – on a games field or athletic track or in a gymnasium.

The sports therapist or coach can exploit this form of resistance more precisely than may at first appear possible. A wide variation in load can be achieved in various ways:

- by altering the resistance with a change of body position
- by the use of partners – either co-operatively or competitively
- by using simple equipment or apparatus.

The exercises shown in Figure 7.8 demonstrate how variation and differences in resistance can be introduced into simple exercises. The two basic exercises here are the press up and the sit up, but the same approach can be used with any body resistance exercise. A useful range of exercises can be achieved working with a partner (Figure 7.9).

Another category of exercises requires gymnasium equipment such as bars, ropes, beams, parallel and wall bars, but still uses the body as the resistance (Figure 7.10).

Very basic aids can be of great use. Get your performer to try the deceptively simple exercise of static sitting, shown in Figure 7.11.

Resistance exercises can prove effective for various types of strength work during normal training, injury avoidance or in the rehabilitation of an injury. They can all be used within minimal space and almost anywhere. Consideration should be given to the type of exercise used, the effects required, the amount and nature of the resistance, the number of repetitions used and the quality of the movements.

Free weights

Since most sports involve the major muscle groups of the body, a basic weight training programme should contain a nucleus of exercises which develop these groups. Onto this basis the specific strength requirements of the sport are added.

Multistation units

The universal or 'multi' gym provides a wide range of exercises while offering some degree of comfort and assistance with the learning of technique. Many single-unit exercise stations have been developed, and most health and fitness clubs have at least some of these. Their design allows a quick and easy change of resistance, and certain exercise

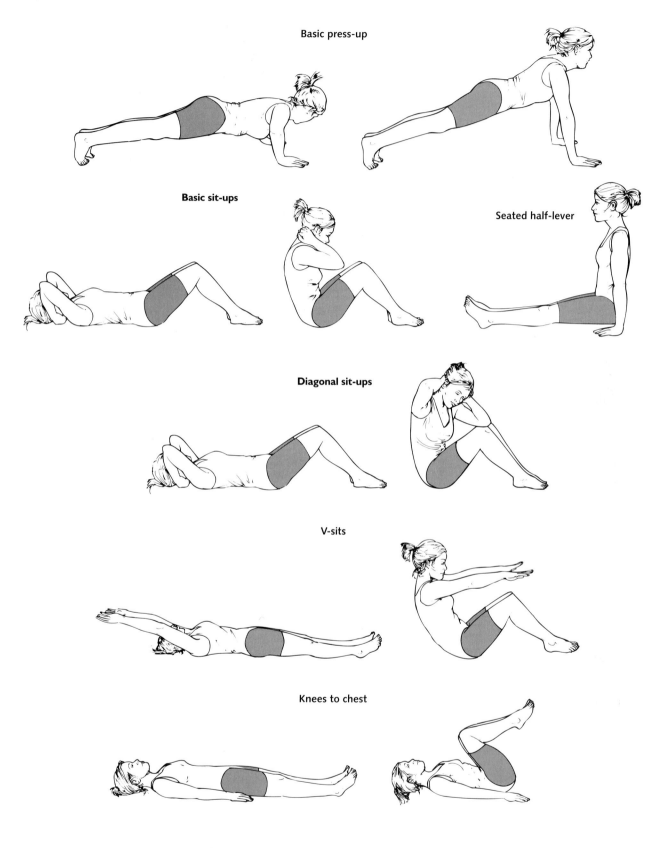

Figure 7.8 *Individual exercises using body resistance*

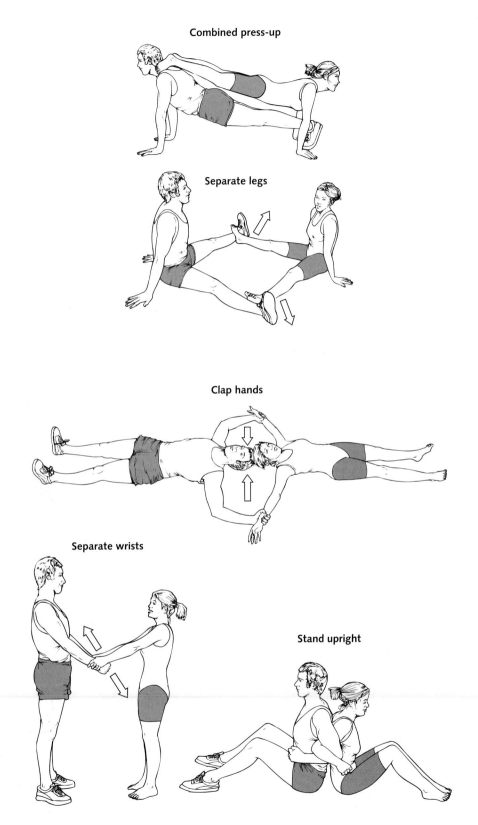

Figure 7.9   *Resistance exercises with a partner*

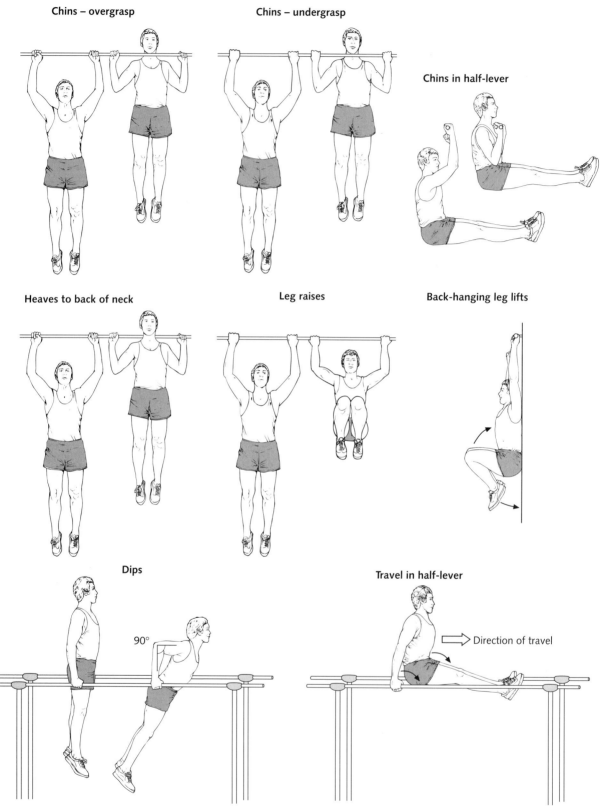

Figure 7.10 *Resistance exercises with equipment*

stations incorporate a variable resistance mode. This book is not the place to instruct you in the use of these machines. The best way is to use a regular set of equipment and make sure that you have been taught how to use each piece correctly.

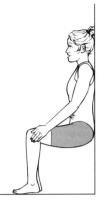

Figure 7.11   Static sitting against a wall

Isometric training

Isometrics involve muscular contractions performed against an immovable resistance. A typical programme to increase strength requires exercises five days a week, during which contractions are held for six seconds at two-thirds of maximum strength. Strength-development isometric training tends to be greatest at the joint angle at which the exercise is performed: if strength is required over a full range of movement then exercises must be performed at several different angles. Many sports require isometric strength and endurance. Obvious examples include wrestling – where strength is required to resist or reposition the opponent – and gymnastics, where the gymnast is required to balance and sustain certain body positions.

Isokinetic training

One of the features of isokinetic training is that the speed of movement may be controlled during the exercise. This is a valuable training factor since most sports muscular force is applied during movement at various speeds. A limb speed close to that used in a particular sport (e.g. the arm action of front crawl) can be preset, allowing the performer to exert optimal force at each point throughout the entire range of the movement on each repetition.

Plyometrics

Plyometrics are training drills that are designed to develop the quality in the athlete which bridges the gap between sheer strength and the power required to produce the explosive muscular movements needed in many sports. In plyometric training the exercise cause a rapid loading of the muscle just before its contraction.

The more a muscle is prestretched from its natural length in the body before its contraction, the greater the load it will be able to lift. In other words, concentric contraction of a muscle (shortening) is much stronger if it immediately follows eccentric contraction (lengthening or prestretching) of the same muscle. There are a number of neuromuscular processes involved, and one possible factor is that at the end of the eccentric phase (the prestretching) energy is stored in the 'elastic' elements of the muscle. This is similar to the way a rubber band snaps back most powerfully when stretched almost to its limit. However, the muscle differs from the rubber band in that the speed of the stretch is an important factor: the faster a muscle is forced to lengthen the greater the tension it exerts, and the rate of stretch is more important that the magnitude of the stretch. Plyometric exercises are used to train this eccentric aspect of muscle action. When designing plyometric exercises remember that maximum tension develops when active muscle is stretched quickly.

PROGRESS CHECK   What is isometric training, and how does it differ from isokinetic training?

Depth jump

Place a pair of boxes or platforms about 1 m apart, with a mat on the floor between them. Keeping the feet together, and emphasising knee flexing, jump from one box to the ground and up onto the other repeatedly (Figure 7.12).

Hurdle spring

Simply make repeated jumps over a single hurdle or a series of hurdles, keeping the feet together and flexing the knees through as large an angle as possible between jumps (Figure 7.13).

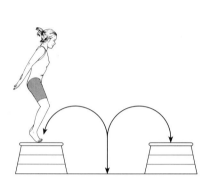

Figure 7.12   *Depth jump*

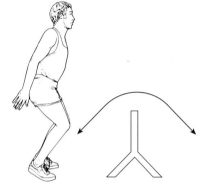

Figure 7.13   *Hurdle spring*

REMEMBER

It is important to test for equipment safety, for exercise appropriateness, and for any contraindications to exercise.

Pulleys and springs

Pulleys allow the direction of a force to be changed so that it is applied at a different angle. This allows you to select a more precise and effective force to suit a given movement. Multi-station units containing pulleys are particularly versatile in this respect, as are appliances in which springs can be extended or compressed so that they can be used either to resist or to assist muscular contraction.

Effects of a strength training programme

Physiological changes accompanying increased strength

There is a relationship between the strength of a muscle and its cross-sectional area. Strength gains are usually accompanied by an increase in the size of individual muscle fibres. This takes the form of an increase in their diameter (muscular hypertrophy). It may be attributed to one or more of the following changes:

- Increase in the numbers and size of the myofibrils.
- Increased amounts of contractile protein, particularly in the myosin filament.
- Increased amounts and strength of connective tendons and ligaments.
- Increased capillary density per fibre.

Increases in strength may also result from improvements in the nervous control of the muscles. Training may, for example, increase the efficiency of the way in which the fibres are selected and recruited to cause an overall muscular contraction.

Assessing the results

Any training programme must be monitored and evaluated regularly to measure its effectiveness. Working progressively through a strength-training programme provides its own intrinsic form of assessment. The known resistances, and the increases in resistances being used, provide regular feedback on improvement. However, if you require separate tests, a few are described here.

Leg press

Sit with the back firmly against the seat, which should be adjusted so that the angle at the knee joint is 90°. With the hands holding the seat rails, press firmly against the pedals and straighten the legs against the resistance until the knee joint is at full extension (Figure 7.14). Note the maximum resistance moved.

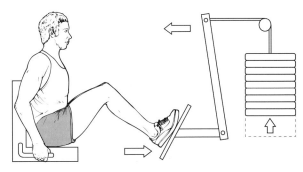

Figure 7.14   *Leg press*

Bench press

Place the bench approximately 5 cm from the weight stack. Lie face up on the bench with your head nearest to the apparatus and feet flat on the floor. Grip the bars, and press against the resistance until the arms are fully extended. Keep the hips in contact with the bench (Figure 7.15). Note the maximum resistance moved.

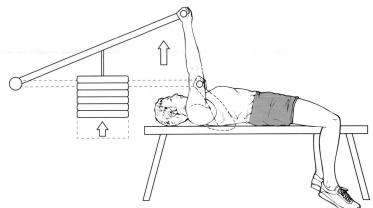

Figure 7.15   *Bench press*

111

Shoulder press

Sit on the stool facing the weight stack, with your back straight. Grip the bars and raise the stack until the arms are fully extended (Figure 7.16). Note the maximum resistance moved.

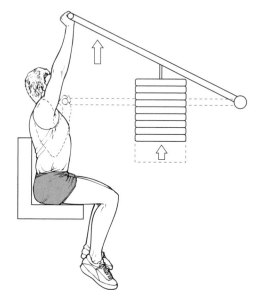

Figure 7.16 *Exercises on a multi-station*

Grip test using hand dynamometer

Use the hand you think is strongest. Place the dynamometer in the palm, dial up, with the needle adjusted so that it points to zero, and grip the bar. Squeeze the dynamometer sharply, as hard as possible, with the arm kept well away from the body (Figure 7.17). Record the best of three attempts. Some people like to raise their arm to shoulder height on the squeeze, others like to lower their arm from shoulder height on the squeeze. It really doesn't matter – as long as you test in exactly the same way every time.

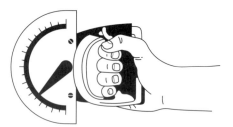

Figure 7.17 *Use of the dynamometer*

Blood pressure

These days the old-fashioned (and some still say superior) sphygmomanometer is not as popular as fully automatic blood pressure units. These are simple to use following the manufacturer's directions. Normal blood pressure is 120 mmHg (systolic), 80 mmHg (diastolic).

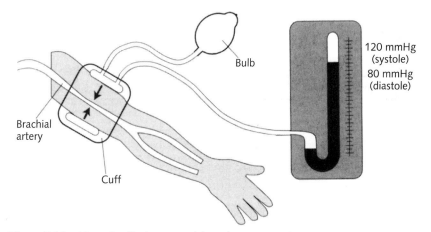

Bulb

120 mmHg
(systole)
80 mmHg
(diastole)

Brachial
artery

Cuff

Figure 7.18 *Measuring blood pressure with a sphygmomanometer*

When testing someone's fitness it is very important to know the demands of the sport for which the athlete is being tested. Your testing programme should be individually designed to accommodate each athlete's requirements.

KEY TERMS

You need to know what these words mean. Go back through the chapter or check the glossary to find out.

Preventive	Protective	Cardiovascular
Warm-up	Progressive	Stretching

---

8 Common sporting injuries

After working through this chapter you will be able to:
➤ assess a patient using the appropriate techniques
➤ identify a common injury
➤ advise a patient as to the cause of their injury
➤ advise on methods of avoiding such an injury
➤ plan treatment and rehabilitation as appropriate.

Before we look at individual injuries, we should spend a little time looking at the type of injury a sports therapist is likely to encounter. In reality the variety is small and the type of treatments available pretty much the same (in the initial stage) for all. Only when we get beyond the first 48 hours does the treatment/rehabilitation go its own way.

Types of injury

Most sports injuries fall into a few general categories. If you understand the treatment and rehabilitation of these injuries you will undoubtedly become a successful practitioner.

Muscular injuries

Muscles are injured either directly, such as by an external blow or force, or by continual repetitive stress from exercise causing **microtrauma** to either a muscle or the musculotendinous unit. Several reasons have been suggested as predisposing factors in muscular injury.

> **microtrauma**
> *minor, insignificant injury which, if occurring repeatedly, will give rise to an obvious injury*

Inadequate warm-up

It is essential that the athlete stretches the muscle to its fullest before training or competing. One of the aims of the warm-up is to gain full flexibility of the muscles, and prevent an injury occurring in the first few minutes of the game or the first few metres of the sprint race because of inadequate flexibility. It is also important to keep warm and flexible during the game, as on a cold day the muscles may tighten again, particularly during a rest break or during a quiet period of the game.

Inadequate fitness

Another group of muscular injuries will occur at the end of the race or game when extra strength, power and endurance may be called for. Other fitness parameters such as flexibility and co-ordination must also be adequate.

Muscle imbalance

Another reason for muscular injury may be an imbalance in the strength/power ratio between the anterior and posterior or medial and lateral muscles. Various ratios have been suggested, but the correct ratio for an individual is probably specific to the demands put on the athlete by the sport in which they are competing. Therefore, a co-ordinated resistance training programme should be carried out on both groups of muscles, to prevent unevenness in speed of muscle contraction and possible muscle strain.

Haematoma

All muscle injuries, no matter what the cause, generally result in haematoma. However, in sports medicine, a haematoma classically refers to an injury caused by direct violence. A haematoma is also known as a contusion. It results from a blow or some external violence to a muscle, typically an opponent's knee hitting the player's quadriceps. This violence causes damage primarily to the blood vessels, and blood seeps into the surrounding tissues. There is generally only minor damage to the muscle tissue itself, although the full extent of the injury will depend on the force of the blow and the state of preparedness of the injured muscle (whether relaxed or contracted) during the impact; the stronger the contraction the less severe the damage.

PROGRESS CHECK

Why would this be the case?

intramuscular
contained within a muscle

intermuscular
between or among muscles; not within one muscle

Another factor that can determine the amount of bleeding is the amount of blood in the area at the time of impact. The more strenuous the effort, the more blood could be expected to be pumped to the muscle to aid performance. This may lead to **intramuscular** or **intermuscular** bleeding, or both.

PROGRESS CHECK

- Muscles are generally injured in two ways: what are they?
- What are the likely predisposing factors in muscular injury?
- What is a haematoma?

Diagnosis

People will generally know if they have been hit although occasionally, in the heat of the moment and with adrenaline pumping, minor knocks are not always noticed. There will be pain, either at rest or on movement with palpation, and often associated protective muscle spasm. Swelling usually occurs within a few hours and, depending on the extent of the injury, bruising (ecchymosis) becomes visible.

heterotopic
occurring in the wrong part of the body

A significant deep haematoma which is neglected may harden and calcify, forming **heterotopic** bone, commonly called myositis ossificans. This hard, egg-shaped mass in the muscle bulk will also form if the injury is pushed too hard in the early stages, preventing full mobility of the limb.

In rare cases, surgery may be needed to remove this calcification but usually, after about 6 weeks of rest, the muscle will return to full function if you follow the correct treatment plan.

Treatment of muscular injuries

Immediate
ICER, as described in Chapter 4. Massage has no place in this early stage – probing fingers could increase the damage to torn blood vessels.

Late treatment
The important aims of late treatment are to regain full muscle extensibility, strength, power and endurance and to regain full function specifically related to the patient's sport.

Exercises should be commenced after application of heat to aid extensibility and muscle contractility. Because of natural weakness in the healing scar tissue of the damaged area and because of the role of the muscles in maintaining joint stability, it is important to begin a gradual progressive overload resistance programme as soon as pain and swelling permit.

PROGRESS CHECK

- What is the difference between inter and intramolecular?
- Describe the routine treatment of a muscle injury, from the injury through to late treatment.

Strain

A muscle usually strains when it is tired or asked to do something suddenly and hasn't been properly prepared for the movement.

Diagnosis
The patient generally says they felt something 'go' and will complain of pain anywhere along the line of the muscle. The muscle is generally very painful on palpation, particularly over the musculotendinous junction. There may also be some pain on stretching the muscle.

Early treatment
The ICER regime will help to ease the pain and spasm and control any swelling or bleeding. A crepe bandage may give some support.

Late treatment
With all muscle injuries the important aim is to prevent the healing scar from limiting normal movement, so stretching exercises should begin as soon as possible, within the limits of pain. An overload weight-training course should be started to ensure that the injured unit regains strength and endurance.

Sprain

A sprain happens to a ligament, usually when the ligament is overstretched or the joint to which it is attached is forced beyond its natural range of movement.

Groin pain

Many patients will present with a condition loosely labelled as 'groin pain'. The condition occurs most frequently in sprinting sports and sports which require great rotational forces at the hips, such as soccer, hockey, jumping events and rugby. The pain may be brought on suddenly by a particular single event or insidiously by continued repetitive movements causing microtrauma over a period of time.

As a variety of structures may be involved or damaged (Figure 8.1), it is vital to carry out a careful examination. A differential diagnosis must consider the following muscles and their tendons, attachments and associated joints:

● iliopsoas (psoas and iliacus)
● rectus femoris
● adductor group
● the pubic symphysis.

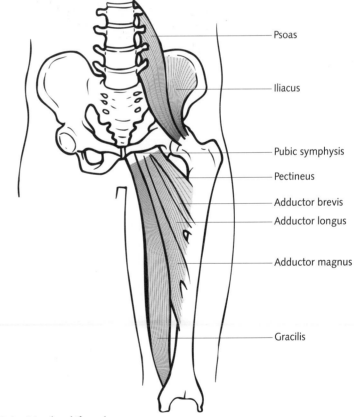

Psoas
Iliacus
Pubic symphysis
Pectineus
Adductor brevis
Adductor longus
Adductor magnus
Gracilis

Figure 8.1 *Muscles of the groin area*

The two most common groin injuries are to the adductor group and the pubic symphysis (osteitis pubis).

117

Adductor muscle strain

Damage to the adductor muscle group typically strikes people who have to sprint and who are required to change direction suddenly while running, such as soccer and hockey players. As contact sports have become more aggressive and dynamic, injury to this muscle group is now common. The primary action of the adductor muscle group is to drag the leg towards the midline of the body – for example, when the leg is swung across the body as in striking a ball. It also stabilises the leg on the pelvis while the pelvis and other leg rotate, as in changing direction. Sudden swerving actions, and propping actions in this direction, often overload the muscles and a strain generally occurs in the muscle bulk of the tendinous attachment of the bone.

The adductor muscle group has a secondary action of assisting the hip while it is flexing and extending, as in lifting the thigh forwards and backwards. Consequently, when great speed is required, the adductor muscle group assists the action which can overload the group and cause damage. This is very much the case with track sprinters and speed athletes.

Diagnosis

An understanding of the biomechanics of this injury is important, so a careful history must be taken, particularly in relation to the player's movements and the location of the pain. As groin pain may also be referred from various orthopaedic conditions of the hip, sacrum and lower back, a thorough assessment of these areas should be undertaken. Other structures which may give groin pain are the rectus femoris, the sacroiliac joint, the iliopsoas and the pubic symphysis.

To test for adductor group strain, the athlete must sit or lie with knees bent and legs apart (hips fully abducted). He or she is then asked to squeeze the legs together (into adduction), against the operator's resistance. This will cause a painful response if there is an adductor muscle strain.

Osteitis pubis

Traumatic osteitis pubis is a stress injury of the symphysis pubis. It is common in soccer players, particularly those participating at a high level. Other athletes who seem to be troubled by the condition are track and field competitors in the disciplines of triple jump, long jump and hurdles, distance runners and rugby players.

Athletes affected with this condition will complain of a combination of the following symptoms:

- an aching pain in the groin radiating down the inside of the leg, sometimes bilaterally
- lower abdominal pain spreading across the anterior abdominal wall
- testicular pain which may also be bilateral; sexual function is often hampered.

History

Patients usually experience increasing groin and abdominal pain over many weeks. The pain will become severe during or some hours after competition and then gradually subside over the next few days. A common pattern is that the athlete competes at the weekend, which induces the pain. The symptoms then gradually subside and by mid-week the athlete can train lightly, and is thus available for the next weekend's competition. This pattern continues until sports performance is affected and the pain becomes so severe that assistance is sought.

Mechanism of injury

An external force applied to the end of the limb produces a shearing stress to the symphysis pubis. The sacroiliac and lumbar spine joints are often involved (Figure 8.2).

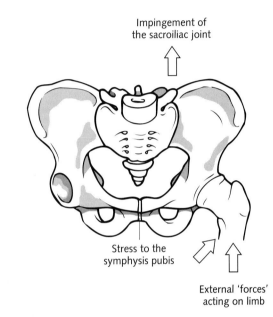

Figure 8.2 *Mechanism of injury in osteitis pubis*

The injury is often a result of overuse, in which microtrauma or repetitive overloading eventually leads to the clinical presentation. In some cases, one traumatic incident, such as a scrum collapse, can precipitate the condition.

Examination

The basis of examination (shown in Figure 8.3) is to differentiate between traumatic osteitis pubis and the adductor muscle strain.

The lumbar spine, hip joints and sacroiliac joints should also be tested, as a strain of these joints and their associated structures can also be present.

Treatment/management

The only treatment of choice in the acute phase is rest from all pain-producing activity. Symptomatic relief can be administered in the form of ice and electrotherapy modalities, such as TENS or ultrasound.

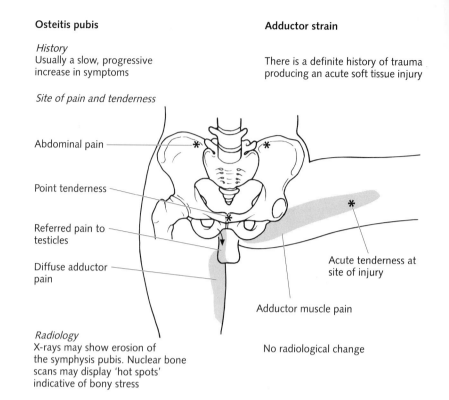

Osteitis pubis

History
Usually a slow, progressive
increase in symptoms

Site of pain and tenderness

Abdominal pain

Point tenderness

Referred pain to
testicles

Diffuse adductor
pain

Radiology
X-rays may show erosion of
the symphysis pubis. Nuclear bone
scans may display 'hot spots'
indicative of bony stress

Adductor strain

There is a definite history of trauma
producing an acute soft tissue injury

Acute tenderness at
site of injury

Adductor muscle pain

No radiological change

Figure 8.3 *Differentiation of traumatic osteitis pubis from an adductor muscle strain (from R.N. Dunn, Traumatic osteitis pubis, Australian Journal of Physiotherapy, 1986, vol. 32, no. 1)*

Rehabilitation

A reduced activity period (approximately 4–6 weeks) is usually necessary to achieve a pain-free state. The athlete should be released by the sports therapist only once they are symptom free. The most common finding is lack of muscle flexibility in the adductors, hip flexors, hamstrings and the erector spinae. A lack of flexibility in these muscle groups is probably a predisposing factor to this injury.

The rehabilitation programme should include comprehensive passive stretching and stretching exercises for the tight muscle groups. Isotonic and isokinetic muscle strengthening routines should be given to all muscles stabilising the pelvis, especially the abdominals, hip extensors and back extensors. Examples of these exercises and further advice on developing a rehabilitation programme can be found in Chapter 7.

PROGRESS CHECK
- Explain the mechanism of adductor muscle strain.
- Explain osteitis pubis.

Calf muscle strain

The calf muscle incorporates the gastrocnemius, the soleus and the Achilles tendon (Figure 8.4).

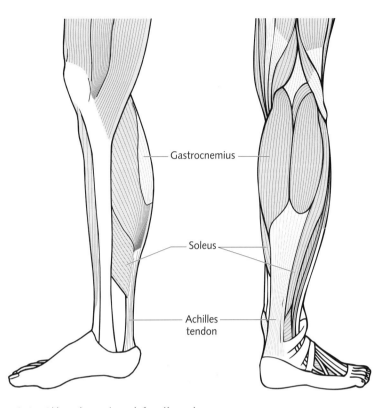

Figure 8.4 *Side and rear views of the calf muscle group*

Damage to any of these structures occurs typically in running and jumping sports, but most injuries are suffered by the 30–40-year-old squash or tennis player.

Diagnosis

The player generally feels as if the calf muscle has been hit from behind by another player and hears a loud snap as the muscle fibres tear. The damage usually occurs at the junction of the medial head of the gastrocnemius and the Achilles tendon. The injured player may collapse in pain and can take no further part in the game.

It is important to differentiate between a muscle strain and a complete Achilles tendon rupture. The Achilles tendon's prime function is to plantar flex the foot (allow it to point down). However, even if the tendon is completely torn, it may still be possible for the athlete to perform the function because the other plantar flexor muscles (the posterior tibial, peroneal and toe flexors) can continue to achieve this action. The Thompson squeeze test (Figure 8.5) is valuable in correctly diagnosing this injury.

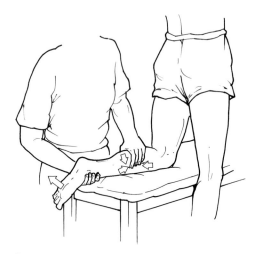

Figure 8.5   *The Thompson squeeze test. With the patient kneeling, foot extended over the edge of the table, squeeze the calf just below the widest part. If the Achilles tendon has lost continuity, the foot will not plantar flex, and the test is positive for a ruptured tendon*

> ── REMEMBER ──
>
> *This injury is greatly influenced by gravity so the leg should be elevated above the level of the heart, on a chair or pillow, and a compression bandage applied. The patient may need crutches or a walking stick for the first few days as bearing weight will inflame the condition.*

If the gastrocnemius muscle is strained, there will also be pain on palpation, and local swelling. Eventually, after several days, bruising may track down the course of the leg to the foot, being influenced by the force of gravity. The cause of this injury is the same as that of other muscular injuries.

Early treatment

Early treatment is aimed at alleviating pain and spasm and controlling excessive swelling so the principles of ICER (described earlier in this book) are essential for the first 24–48 hours.

Late treatment

As soon as pain permits, exercises should be commenced to regain normal muscle flexibility and the other components of strength and fitness. The aim is to stretch and strengthen the healing tissue, building up to normal function.

PROGRESS CHECK

- Explain the mechanism of a calf muscle strain.

Knee injuries

The knee joint is a complex yet stable modified hinge joint, well developed by evolution to function very efficiently in normal circumstances. Unlike other mammals (except elephants), humans have the distinction of bearing weight upon this joint in extension, instead of in the flexed position which acts as a shock absorber for other species. This renders the joint very vulnerable, as the stresses placed upon it by extreme athletic pursuits make the incidence of knee injury very high among people playing sport.

Anatomy of the knee

To be able to localise a particular condition, it will be necessary to revise certain aspects of the functional anatomy of the knee. The knee is not a simple hinge joint. It is bicondylar, which allows the tibia to rotate in its longitudinal axis to various degrees of flexion with maximal rotation occurring at 90° of flexion. No rotation occurs in full extension (Figure 8.6).

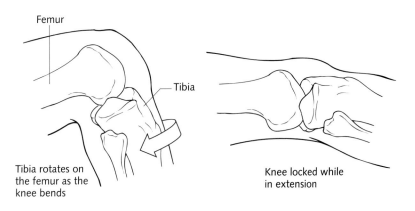

Femur

Tibia

Tibia rotates on the femur as the knee bends

Knee locked while in extension

Figure 8.6   *The tibia rotates as the knee bends*

The stability of the knee depends primarily on muscular support and on the action of the cruciate and collateral ligaments, and to a lesser extent, the menisci (cartilages). The collateral ligaments (medial and lateral) are responsible for transverse stability during knee extension and the cruciates and collaterals together are responsible for anteroposterior (forward and backward) stability, allowing the joint to work as a hinge.

During walking and running, the knee may be subjected to abnormal stresses. If these stresses are too severe, a particular structure or structures will be damaged.

Diagnosis

Anyone who is responsible at any level for the care of athletes should know how to carry out a meaningful examination of a knee injury. It is sometimes possible to diagnose the exact damage to a knee if it is examined within half an hour after injury – before the reactions of inflammation, pain and swelling limit movement for diagnostic purposes.

123

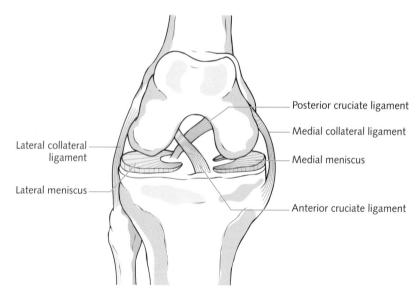

Figure 8.7 *The normal knee joint*

History

In many traumatic conditions of the knee, the diagnosis may depend on the history alone. Thus the importance of taking a thorough history cannot be overstressed. The development of symptoms is traced step by step from their beginnings to the time of consultation. The patient's assessment of how the condition or injury occurred, and even an onlooker's interpretation of the event, can be very useful.

Diagnosis of ligament injuries

Medial collateral ligament

The most common injury to the knee is damage to the medial collateral ligament, generally caused by a blow to the outside of the knee causing stress on the inside (Figure 8.8).

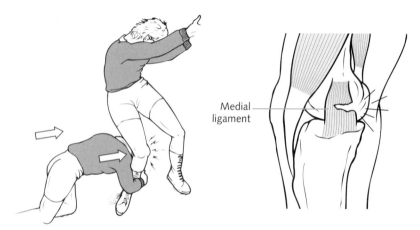

Figure 8.8 *Action causing damage to the medial ligament*

Medial ligament sprain is tested with the knee in complete extension and at 30° flexion. Inward pressure is applied on the outside of the knee while the ankle is supported. This will produce pain on the inside of the knee, generally at the attachment of the medial ligament to the femur or tibia (Figure 8.9).

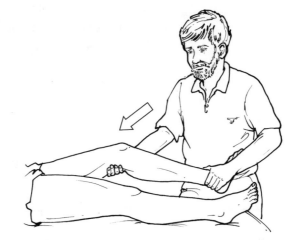

Figure 8.9 *Testing for medial ligament damage*

The test for lateral ligament damage is the reverse of that for the medial ligament: outward pressure is applied to the femur on the inside of the leg while supporting the ankle.

Cruciate ligaments

The cruciate ligaments lie in the centre of the joint, crossing each other (hence the name: cruciate means 'cross shaped'). They are mainly responsible for backwards and forwards stability. The simplest way to damage one or both of these ligaments is to fall on the front part of the tibia (Figure 8.10).

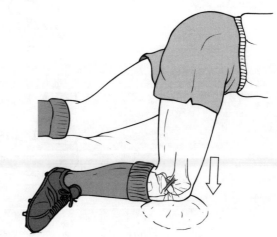

Figure 8.10 *Injury to the cruciate ligaments*

A lesion (injury) of the posterior cruciate ligament leads to a posterior (backwards) displacement. Similarly, a lesion of the anterior cruciate leads to abnormal anterior (forward) displacement.

There are three tests for anterior cruciate ligament damage:

- the Lachman test (Figure 8.11)
- the anterior draw test (Figure 8.12)
- the crossover test (Figure 8.13).

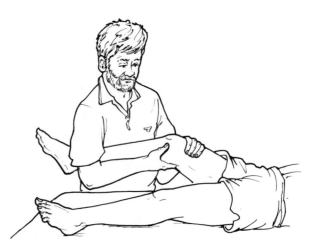

Figure 8.11   *The Lachman test*

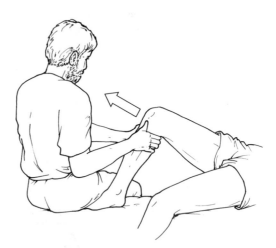

Figure 8.12   *The anterior draw test. With the knee bent at 90°, test for excessive movement of the tibia forwards in relation to the femur.*

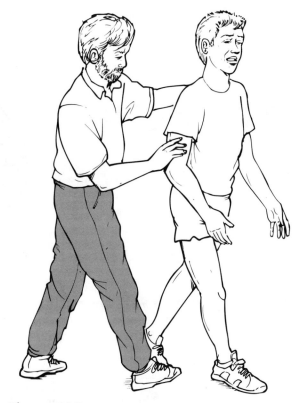

Figure 8.13 *The crossover test*

Posterior cruciate ligament testing is usually the opposite to the anterior draw test, and is most often a reliable indication of posterior cruciate damage.

Cartilage injury

Occasionally, if the cartilage is torn and the torn shred resumes its original position (and function), no treatment may be necessary except routine pain relief and appropriate exercise. However, although the joint may be symptom free for years, the torn cartilage can be displaced by a relatively simple rotary movement on the flexed knee (Figure 8.14). If the joint becomes continually painful and swollen, and if it locks or 'gives way' regularly, strong consideration should be given for the meniscus, or part thereof, to be removed.

Fluid and effusion are not always reliable guides to severity of a meniscus injury. Neither is pain, as only damage of peripheral structures will register pain.

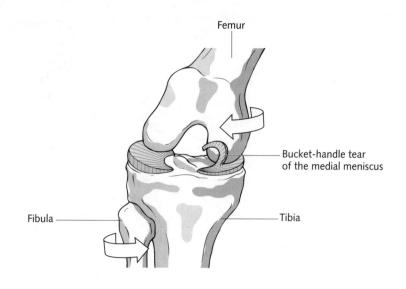

Figure 8.14 *Cartilage injury: the knee is bent and the femur is rotating on the tibia, causing a tearing of the medial meniscus*

The McMurray test

There are many variations of this test and experience is needed for its results to be meaningful. The knee should be bent to the greatest amount of flexion possible and the fingers and thumb placed over the joint line to detect 'clicks' and 'clunks' as the tibia is rotated to extremes on the femur (Figure 8.15).

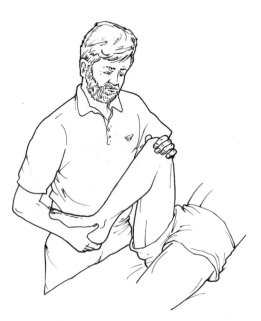

Figure 8.15 *The McMurray test*

The knee should flex past 90° for the test to be useful. When positive, with good 'clunks' resounding, the test is very helpful. When negative, it means little.

Damage to bursae and synovial membranes

Overuse or direct violent contact can inflame and damage these structures. There is a local tenderness, swelling and inflammation. Pain is usually present with tension of the skin in extreme flexion or under direct contact pressure.

Treatment of knee injuries

Treatment is virtually the same as for any injury, anywhere in the body. The main objectives are to:

- relieve pain and inflammation
- control swelling
- aid healing
- regain and maintain muscular control of the joint by intensive exercise
- regain the full range of movement and mobility
- regain full function of the joint.

As with all injuries in the early (acute) stage, follow the ICER routine as already discussed. The later stages of treatment/rehabilitation aim to regain strength, mobility, proprioception, power and function.

PROGRESS CHECK

- Explain the anatomy of the knee.
- What part of the knee is the structure most often damaged?
- Where would you find the cruciate liagments, and what are their names?

Ankle injuries

Soft-tissue injuries to the ankle joint are very common among athletes. The lateral ligament is damaged as much as five times as often as the medial ligament. In fact, the lateral ligament complex of the ankle is the most frequently injured single structure in the body. This fact is important in understanding both the mechanism of injury and its prevention. Furthermore, because the ankle is a weight-bearing joint and closely associated with balance, if soft-tissue injuries to this joint are treated incorrectly, or even lightly, the old adage 'once a sprain, always a sprain' may prove correct.

Early and correct management is important and should be followed by a plan specifically suited to the injury. In this way, no soft-tissue ankle injury should be a handicap to any athlete.

Cause

The ankle suffers a sprain when the ligaments are overstretched (Figure 8.16). This occurs most frequently when the foot is inverted, plantar

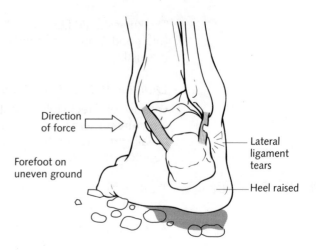

Figure 8.16   A lateral ligament sprain – rear view

flexed and internally rotated, placing the ankle in a most unstable position. A force from any direction with the foot in this situation may damage the ligament and joint capsule.

Diagnosis

At the first possible opportunity, a radiograph should be taken to eliminate any damage to the bone (an ankle fracture is actually a rare occurrence). If squeezing the midshaft of the fibula produces pain at the ankle joint, a fracture may well be present (Figure 8.17).

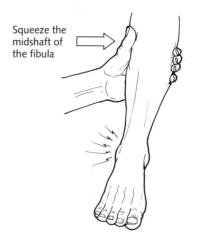

Figure 8.17   Squeeze the midshaft of the fibula to test for possible ankle fractures

After appropriate questioning about the circumstances of the injury, and of the forces involved, it should be easy to determine the site of damage. Observation, plus palpation over the suspected area, will then localise the ligaments concerned. Finally, stress and stability tests should be undertaken to gauge both the severity of damage and any joint instability. The most common one to consider here is the inversion test (Figure 8.18).

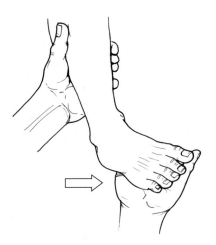

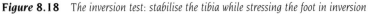

Figure 8.18   *The inversion test: stabilise the tibia while stressing the foot in inversion*

The best time to carry out an examination is as soon as the patient is brought from the field and before severe pain, spasm and swelling limit effective diagnosis.

Treatment

As with all injuries, follow the routine:

- relieve pain and inflammation
- control swelling
- aid healing
- regain and maintain musculature
- regain full range of movement and mobility
- regain full function.

Some very basic ideas for exercises appropriate for the ankle joint are shown in Figure 8.19.

PROGRESS CHECK
- Which ligament of the ankle is most often damaged?
- What causes a sprain?
- How would you treat a sprained ankle?

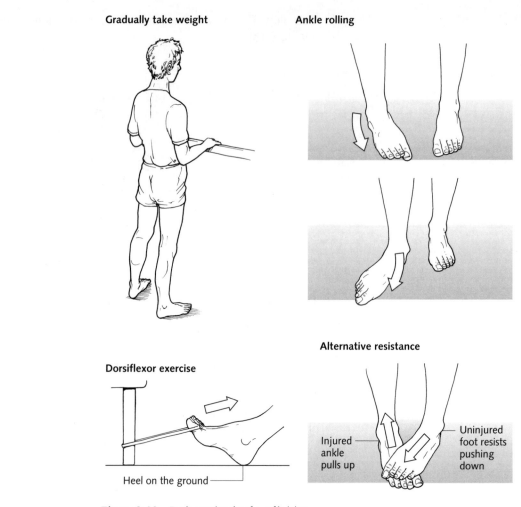

Figure 8.19 *Basic exercises for the ankle joint*

Upper limb injuries

The most common injuries to the upper limb in body contact sport occur to the shoulder girdle and finger (metacarpal joints). Overuse injuries occur also to the elbow and wrist joints.

Shoulder girdle injuries

The most common injuries in this area are

- acromioclavicular joint damage
- sternoclavicular joint damage
- glenohumeral joint dislocation
- rotator cuff impingement syndrome.

The glenohumeral joint is a modified ball and socket joint, which allows for a great range of movement around the shoulder. This great mobility has a trade-off in sport, particularly contact sport, as stability is often compromised. Because of the long levers involved and the many intricate and heavy actions required, the joints of the shoulder girdle are often damaged.

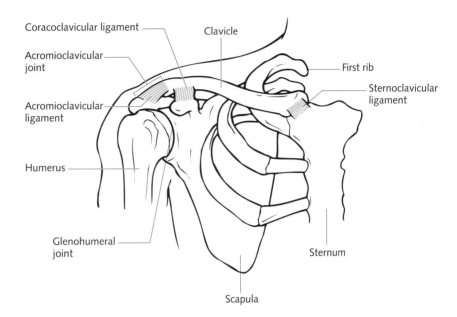

Figure 8.20 *The joints of the shoulder girdle*

Acromioclavicular joint

This is a relatively unstable joint, which is often damaged during contact sports. Injury typically occurs when the point of the shoulder is speared into the ground or into an opposing player or post. It can also be caused by a direct kick or a fall on the outstretched hand. Depending on the extent of the injury, a swelling on top of the shoulder generally results, with pain on touching and limitation in the range of shoulder movement (grade one injury). A grade two sprain will also display damage to the coracoclavicular ligament and the clavicle will be raised slightly in relation to the acromial process. A grade three sprain indicates complete rupture of both the acromioclavicular and coracoclavicular ligaments, and results in very obvious elevation of the clavicle. This injury is particularly prevalent in rugby players, obviously because of the tackling inherent in the game.

Treatment/rehabilitation
Follow the routine that we have already discussed:

- relieve pain and inflammation
- control swelling

- aid healing
- regain and maintain muscle control of the joint by intensive exercise
- regain the full range of movement and mobility
- regain full function.

Sternoclavicular joint

This is not often damaged in sport, as little movement takes place in and around the joint. It anchors the clavicle onto the sternum – and as the clavicle is a stabiliser for the shoulder joint proper, it is mainly injured by violence to this joint or by telescopic action from a fall or tackle on the outstretched arm.

Glenohumeral joint dislocation

The most common of all shoulder joint dislocations is anterior dislocation of the glenohumeral joint. It occurs generally as a result of violent contact with either another player or an obstacle such as the ground or a goalpost. The arm is forced into abduction and externally rotated. Excessive throwing action may also dislocate this joint.

The damage may be quite extensive as the greater tuberosity of the humerus is pushed out of its labrum, perhaps damaging it on the way, plus stretching or tearing the glenohumeral ligament, the anterior joint capsule and possibly also the rotator cuff muscles.

The injury is accompanied by intense pain and an immediate protective muscle spasm of the shoulder girdle muscles.

Immediate treatment

This injury requires immediate medical attention. The shoulder should be packed in ice and the patient allowed to support themselves in the position they find most comfortable (or least uncomfortable). *Under no circumstances* should you attempt to place the shoulder back into its normal position.

Rotator cuff impingement syndrome

Pain around the shoulder joint usually arises from pathology affecting the components of the rotator cuff complex. Painful arc syndrome, rotator cuff tendonitis, supraspinatus tendonitis and bursitis are all used to describe pain and dysfunction of the shoulder originating from soft tissue injury. For the purposes of this book, the term 'rotator cuff impingement syndrome' is used to describe this spectrum of pathological entities.

Anatomy of the rotator cuff

The superficial muscles around the shoulder region (Figure 8.21) are responsible for the gross movements of the shoulder joint. The prime movers, which extend the shoulder backwards, are the latissimus dorsi and the posterior deltoid. Flexing in a forward motion is initiated by the anterior deltoid; all the fibres of the deltoid acting in conjunction will raise the arm outwards from the body (abduction). Pectoralis major moves the arm horizontally across the body and the trapezius will shrug the shoulder girdle.

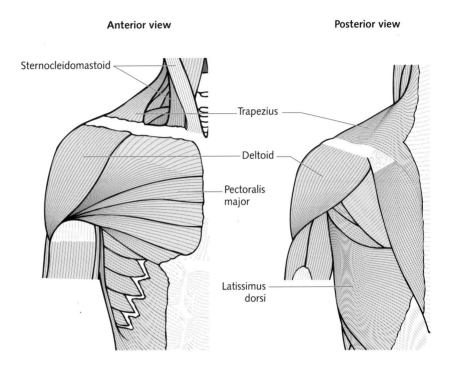

Figure 8.21 *Superficial muscles of the shoulder*

Below the superficial muscles are a deeper group, collectively known as the rotator cuff (Figure 8.22). These muscles are responsible for the intricate movements of the shoulder, such as rotation of the arm during activities such as throwing and swimming. The rotator cuff consists of the following muscles:

- subscapularis
- supraspinatus
- infraspinatus
- teres minor.

Supraspinatus is the primary muscle involved in rotator cuff impingement syndrome. Other structures that also may be involved include the biceps tendon, the subacromial bursa and the joint capsule.

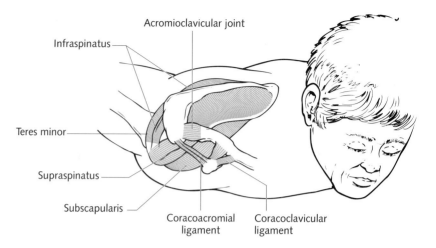

Figure 8.22 *The rotator cuff muscles, viewed from above*

Table 8.1 *Pathology of the rotator cuff impingement syndrome*

Stage	Pathology	Prognosis
1	Irritation leading to swelling and bleeding	Reversible
2	Inflammation of the tendon (tendonitis) and fibrosis (scarring) and thickening	Reversible
3	Degeneration and eventual tearing of the tendon	Often irreversible

Cause of injury

As with all other syndromes, the primary cause is an error in training. Shoulder pain tends to be recurrent in athletes, the symptoms occurring either in the beginning of the season or near the end. This is because athletes are either trying to upgrade their training too quickly or are getting tired as the intensity of training and playing increases.

Incorrect technique also plays a dominant role in injury. The correct throwing style can reduce the stress to shoulder and arm. The whipping action of a side-arm throw may slightly increase the speed of delivery – however, this technique, particularly when the body opens up too soon in the delivery, will cause excessive stress to the upper limb. Overhead strokes, a mishit, or trying to put too much spin on the ball in a tennis serve are common injury-producing situations.

Signs and symptoms

Young competitive athletes normally experience insidious onset of soreness after or during activity. The pain is usually felt below the shoulder joint at the point of insertion of the deltoid (Figure 8.23). The pain increases as the overload activity continues until it interferes with function. In the less fit or unskilled athlete the cause may be one traumatic incident (such as mishitting an overhead smash in tennis), which is painful for some time after the incident. The pain usually subsides in a day or two, only to return at the next attempt at sport. Table 8.2 illustrates the various stages in the development of symptoms.

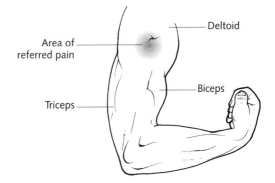

Figure 8.23 *The area where tenderness is usually experienced in rotator cuff impingement*

Table 8.2 *Stages in the development of symptoms in rotator cuff impingement syndrome*

Stage	Symptoms
I	Pain develops after injury
II	Pain begins to occur with activity but the athlete can continue with no decrease in performance
III	The athlete continues to play but pain significantly affects performance
IV	The athlete cannot compete and experiences continued pain, even at rest

Treatment

The treatment of shoulder pain is based on the three major principles consistently discussed throughout this book:

* symptomatic relief
* rehabilitation
* correction of fault.

Elbow joint injuries

The most common injuries to the elbow joint are to the medial and lateral epicondyles. The main cause is overuse.

Tennis elbow

This is a condition that is not only common amongst athletes but also occurs in many vocations. The term itself is misleading as it suggests that only tennis players are susceptible. However, the elbow is notoriously susceptible to injury from any repetitive task. Tennis elbow can be brought about by any activity involving repeated forceful grip, especially if combined with rotation of the forearm, such as using a screwdriver or painting. These activities demand the same action of the forearm muscles as does the tennis stroke. Therefore any occupation, hobby, home task or sport involving the repetition of such movements can cause tennis elbow.

The medical term usually applied to tennis elbow is epicondylitis. It refers to a painful inflammation of the tendons of origin in the forearm muscles; the wrist and finger extensors on the lateral side (lateral epicondylitis) and the wrist and finger flexors on the medial side (medial epicondylitis) (Figure 8.24). Repetitive overload causes microtraumas to these tendons. This damage will lead to inflammation (tendonitis).

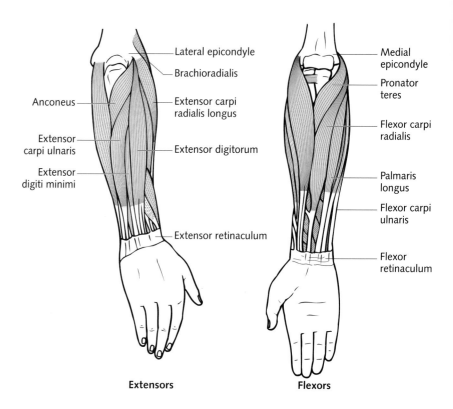

Figure 8.24 *Flexor and extensor muscles of the forearm*

Treatment

The basic treatment approach to tennis elbow is to follow five logical steps:

1   Relieve pain and inflammation.
2   Promote healing.
3   Regain the strength, power, endurance and flexibility of both arm and forearm.
4   Reduce the overload forces to the elbow which caused the injury.
5   Allow gradual return to sport/activity.

As with the treatment of all injuries, if each of these steps is not followed to its conclusion, the treatment will fail.

Wrist and hand injuries

Wrist sprain

Because of the intricate and versatile movements which the wrist allows and the delicacy of the bones and supporting structures which form it, the wrist is often damaged in sport. The most common cause of injury is a fall on the extended or hyperextended wrist. However, excessive jarring

138

from power movements in racquet sports can also overload this joint. The most common injury is a sprain of the anterior or posterior ligaments supporting the wrist.

Signs and symptoms

A sprained wrist will have generalised swelling, point tenderness and limitation of wrist movement, whereas a fractured scaphoid will have almost no swelling, reasonable joint movement and pain on compression of the scaphoid bone. It is possible that both injuries will occur in the same accident, so it is vital to secure a positive diagnosis, as the fractured scaphoid must be immobilised to aid healing and prevent possible complications of malunion and non-union.

The treatment of a wrist sprain follows the classical lines of ICER (see Chapter 4). Exercises for the wrist are shown in Figure 8.25.

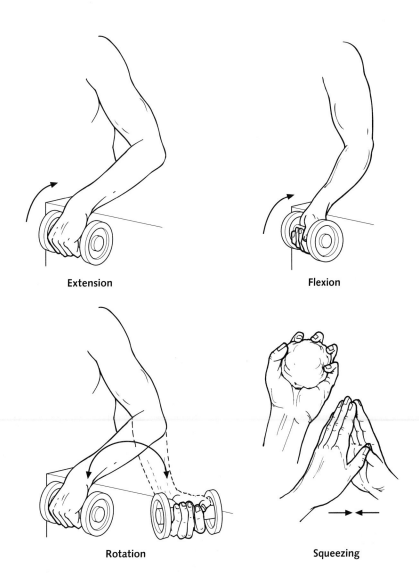

Extension

Flexion

Rotation

Squeezing

Figure 8.25 *Exercises for the wrist*

Injuries to the fingers and thumb

The most common injuries to this region are dislocations, sprains and fractures of the phalanges. All three types of injuries occur from a similar mechanism; external force from a fall, blow or twisting action.

The obvious signs of fractures are deformity, **crepitus** and excessive movement. If these signs are not present and a fracture is suspected because of localised tenderness over the shaft and only a little swelling, a radiograph is necessary. Treatment is mainly by immobilisation by splinting, depending on the extent of damage; always refer to a doctor.

A dislocation of the finger mainly involves damage to the capsular tissue but, because of the extent of damage and the possibility of a small fracture, these injuries should also be checked by a radiograph. Considerable scarring results from this injury and the joint must be mobilised as soon as pain permits. Passive mobilising techniques are very important, as well as resisted exercises to regain normal function and to prevent 'lumpy' swollen phalanx joints.

crepitus

a grating sound or feeling sometimes encountered in fractures, tendonitis and joint injuries

PROGRESS CHECK

- Which muscles make up the rotator cuff?
- Explain the mechanism of a tennis elbow injury.

KEY TERMS

You need to know what these words mean. Go back through the chapter or check the glossary to find out.

Extrinsic	Imbalance	Strain
Intrinsic	Haematoma	Sprain

9

Diet and nutrition for the sports therapist

After working through this chapter you will be able to:
➤ identify the different sources of energy
➤ understand the role each plays
➤ have some understanding of daily nutritional requirements
➤ use the information to assess your own and your athletes' diets.

This chapter will look at the basic principles of nutrition and the link between nutrition and sports performance. Remember, there is no point in improving your knowledge if you do not pass the lessons on.

Energy sources

Originally, all food energy comes from the sun. Plants capture the sun's energy and store it, often in the form of starch. Humans take in this energy either directly by eating the plants themselves or indirectly by eating the meat or byproducts (eggs, milk, etc.) of animals which have consumed the plants.

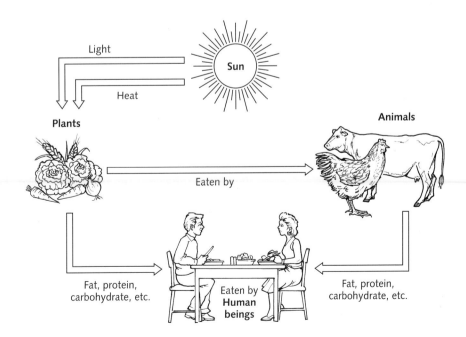

Figure 9.1 *Human energy sources*

ATP

adenosine triphosphate, a form of chemical energy found in all cells. When ATP is broken down to adenosine diphosphate (ADP) and phosphate, energy is released

Our digestive systems break down the nutritious parts of the food into simple sugars and fats. Muscle cells extract energy from these sugars and fats by two different processes, aerobic or anaerobic, depending upon how long and how hard the muscle is working. The aerobic process requires the uptake of oxygen, and consumes both sugars (mainly glucose in its storage from glycogen) and fats. The anaerobic process operates without oxygen, and consumes only the sugars. In both processes the usable proportion of the energy is delivered in the form of **ATP**. This is the basic currency of energy metabolism within the cell, regardless of the source or method by which it is initially generated.

Some definitions

Nutrition

Nutrition is the process by which chemicals from the environment are taken up by the body in order to provide the energy and nutrients needed to keep you alive and healthy.

Diet

A diet can best be described as a particular pattern of eating habits designed to regulate the amount of nutrients consumed.

Food and the recommended intake of nutrients

Food is composed of the following nutrients:

- carbohydrates
- fats
- proteins
- alcohol
- vitamins
- minerals
- trace elements
- dietary fibre
- water.

The amount of these nutrients available varies widely between different foods. As no single food contains enough of each nutrient to meet the body's needs, it is essential to consume a wide variety of foods.

Published tables list the recommended daily intake (RDI) of the various nutrients, according to age, weight, lean body mass, growth, sex and level of activity. These recommendations can be met by taking in a wide variety of foods, and the body can store any nutrient in sufficient quantity to last a few days.

Digestion

Digestion is the process by which the larger chemical compounds within foods are broken down in the gut into smaller compounds so that they may be absorbed by the body.

Absorption

This is the way the nutrients from the digested food move into the body from the stomach and small intestine. The food that is not absorbed passes straight through the body and is eventually excreted – not everything we eat is absorbed.

Excretion

The removal of the end products of metabolism from the body, primarily in urine. Nutrients that have been absorbed by the body are metabolised, and the unwanted by-products are then excreted from the body.

PROGRESS CHECK

- Where does human energy originate from?
- Our digestive systems break down our food into two things – what?
- Define nutrition.

Energy

Almost every function performed by the cells in the body requires energy. The system is constantly converting food into fresh ATP to replace that consumed by the cells.

The energy within food is measured in terms of the amount of heat that would be liberated by its complete breakdown in the body. The old units of energy were Calories (or more correctly kilocalories (kcal)), but we now use joules (J), kilojoules (1 kJ = 1000 joules) or megajoules (1 MJ = 1000 kJ). To convert kilocalories into kilojoules, simply multiply the number of kilocalories by 4.2. The energy in your diet is mainly obtained from the carbohydrates and fat in food, although some comes from protein and alcohol. No energy is provided by vitamins or minerals.

The amount of energy that you require each day depends on many factors, such as:

- your size
- your weight
- how much exercise you do.

The typical energy intake for a man is between 4 and 20 MJ (1000–5000 kcal), the range for a woman is 4–15 MJ (1000–3500 kcal). However, it is not possible to state how much energy a sportsperson needs each day – it will vary considerably between individuals. If you take in more energy than you actually require, the excess will simply be stored as fat and your weight will increase. Similarly, if you do not take in sufficient energy, you will need to call upon your body's stores to meet the demand, and you will lose weight.

Recommended daily intake of energy

The quantities of protein, vitamins, minerals etc. remain broadly proportional in adults. Children and pregnant women need a markedly higher intake of calcium and iron. Lactating mothers also need much more vitamin A.

Table 9.1 *Recommended daily energy intakes*

Age range (years)	Occupational category	Energy requirements	
		kcal	MJ
Girls			
9–12		2300	9.6
12–15		2300	9.6
15–18		2300	9.6
Women			
18–55	Most occupations	2200	9.2
	Very active	2500	10.5
55–75	Assumed sedentary	2050	8.6
75+		1900	8.0
During pregnancy		2400	10.0
(2nd and 3rd trimesters)			
During lactation		2700	11.3
Boys			
9–12		2500	10.5
12–15		2800	11.7
15–18		3000	12.6
Men			
18–35	Sedentary	2700	11.3
	Moderately active	3000	12.6
	Very active	3600	15.1
35–65	Sedentary	2600	10.9
	Moderately active	2900	12.1
	Very active	3600	15.1
65–75	Assumed sedentary	2350	9.8
75+		2100	8.8

PROGRESS CHECK

- Food is composed of which nutrients?
- Explain digestion
- What is meant by absorption?
- What factors decide the amounts of energy we need each day?

The constituents of food and drink

Carbohydrates

Carbohydrates are composed of only carbon, hydrogen and oxygen. Their basic unit is simple sugar or monosaccharide, the most common of which occurring in food is glucose.

The best types of high-carbohydrate foods are those containing carbohydrates in their natural, unrefined state (complex carbohydrates), mainly as starch in whole grains and grain produce. The best examples are high-fibre foods which have been subjected to the minimum of processing, such as:

- wholemeal bread
- wholemeal pasta
- cereal

- pulses and legumes (peas and beans)
- vegetables and nuts.

Highly processed foods can be high in simple carbohydrates (carbohydrates that have been extracted and broken down into relatively simple disaccharides), which can then be rapidly absorbed following minimal digestion. Typical examples are:

- sweet foods such as sugar
- preserves
- confectionery.

Although these foods are quite high in carbohydrate, they usually contain either relatively small amounts of other nutrients or lots of fat. Therefore they are considered to be less nutritious than the less-processed foods containing complex carbohydrate.

Carbohydrates help to maintain the energy stores of the body (as glycogen) and are used in the synthesis of important compounds in the body. A typical daily carbohydrate intake for a man in the UK is 250–350 g; a woman would consume around 150–300 g per day. This provides 40–45% of the total energy in the diet. Recent research suggests that it could be beneficial to increase this proportion to at least 50%.

Fats

triglyceride

the basic component of a fat, consisting of three fatty acids attached to a glycerol backbone

Fats are also composed of carbon, hydrogen and oxygen; although the proportion of oxygen is less than in carbohydrate. The basic component of fat is the **triglyceride**.

During digestion triglycerides are broken down into their constituent fatty acids and glycerol, which can then be absorbed. Fats are important nutrients, not only as a source of energy but also to synthesise many important compounds and tissues vital for normal functioning. However, it is generally believed that we eat far too much fat in our diet, particularly the saturated fats. Even though fat provides much of the flavour, colour and texture in our foods, a low-fat diet does not have to be unpalatable.

A typical daily fat intake is 100–150 g for men and 75–130 g for women. Fats provide 40–45% of the total energy in the diet. The latest recommendations suggest that this proportion is too high, and that we should reduce it to no more than 35–40%.

Proteins

essential amino acid

an amino acid that is needed for protein synthesis but which we cannot make ourselves and must therefore take in in the diet

Proteins are large molecules which the digestive system breaks down into simple units called amino acids. These contain hydrogen, oxygen, nitrogen and in some cases sulphur. There are 21 different amino acids, but they can be combined together with almost infinite variety.

Foods containing high amounts of **essential amino acids** are:

- meat
- fish and
- dairy produce

although the contribution made by non-animal sources such as

- cereals
- legumes
- pulses and
- nuts

should not be overlooked.

The traditional view of 'first class' (animal) and 'second class' (vegetable) proteins is not strictly true. It stems from the mistaken belief that the protein found in plants is of inferior quality to that in meat. Vegetable proteins *do* contain essential amino acids, simply in smaller quantities than those in animal proteins. This deficiency can be overcome by eating plenty of different types of vegetable protein. Combining vegetable protein low in one particular essential amino acid with another high in that amino acid results in a protein of reasonable quality.

Men typically take in up to 100 g protein a day, women 75 g per day. Protein provides 10–15% of the total energy intake.

Vitamins

Vitamins are chemical compounds needed by the body in minute amounts to perform specific functions. In general they cannot be made by the body, and so must be obtained from the diet.

Obvious signs of vitamin deficiency in either the general public or sportspeople are now rare. However, the possibility that low vitamin levels in the body may impair performance should not be overlooked.

Minerals, electrolytes and trace elements

Your body requires:

- iron
- sodium
- potassium
- calcium
- phosphorus and
- magnesium

in very small amounts.

Excess consumption of some minerals, particularly when taken as supplements, can result in a toxic accumulation which may be harmful. A typical example is iron.

Fibre

Fibre is basically non-digestible carbohydrate material which forms the skeleton of plants. It is not actually absorbed by the body and is often ignored when considering nutrients. However, it is vitally important. It adds bulk to the food as it passes through the body, is essential to the proper functioning of the gut, and is thought to assist in the absorption of minerals.

Table 9.2 *Vitamins*

Vitamin	Sources	Involved in
A (retinol; carotene)	Liver, dairy produce, eggs, carrots, green leafy vegetables	Vision, skin, connective tissue
B_1 (thiamin)	Meat, whole grains, legumes, nuts	Carbohydrate metabolism, CNS* function
B_2 (riboflavin)	Liver, dairy produce, meat, cereal products	Carbohydrate metabolism, skin, vision
B_6 (pyridoxine)	Meat, fish, green leafy vegetables, whole grains, legumes	Protein metabolism, formation of red blood cells, CNS function
B_{12} (cyanocobalamin)	Meat, fish, dairy produce: no vegetable sources	Formation of red blood cells, CNS function
Niacin	Liver, meat, fish, cereal products	Carbohydrate metabolism, fat metabolism
Folic acid	Liver, legumes, green leafy vegetables	Regulates growth of cells, including red blood cells
C (ascorbic acid)	Green leafy vegetables, fruit, potatoes, white bread	Connective tissue, iron absorption/metabolism, healing/control of infection
D (calciferol)	Dairy produce, action of sunlight on the skin	Calcium metabolism, bones and teeth
E (tocopherol)	Vegetable oils, liver, green leafy vegetables, dairy and produce, whole grains	Protects vitamins A and C fatty acids from destruction in the body (anti-oxidant)

*Central nervous system

A typical fibre intake is about 15–25 g per day for both men and women. This is now considered to be too low. Of course it is possible to go to the other extreme and it should be remembered that excessive fibre consumption also has its dangers – as with all aspects of diet, it is balance which is important.

Water

Water is one of the most important substances. It is the main means of transport within the body, conveying nutrients, waste metabolites and internal secretions (e.g. hormones) to their target tissues. It holds oxygen and carbon dioxide in solution, as well as hydrogen ions, the concentration of which determines the blood's acidity level. Water is also the prime component of many cells – and because it is a powerful ionising agent it controls the distribution of numerous electrolytes, both within cells and throughout the body.

The role water plays in the regulation of the body's temperature is of vital importance, particularly during exercise. It performs this function in two ways:

1 the water within the cells absorbs heat generated there during energy liberation and transports it to the skin for eventual dissipation

2 when excreted as sweat, it evaporates, which has a cooling effect on the body.

Even small losses of water (2–3% of body weight) can seriously impair performance.

PROGRESS CHECK

- Give three examples each of: carbohydrates, fats, proteins, vitamins, minerals.
- What role does fibre play in the body?
- Why do we need water?

Alcohol

Alcohol is the product of the fermentation of carbohydrate by yeasts; it should make only a minor contribution to your total energy intake. Alcohol differs from carbohydrate and fat in that it cannot be used by the muscles to provide energy during exercise. Furthermore, it cannot be used to provide a rapid release of energy on demand, as it is slowly metabolised by the liver at a constant rate. Therefore any energy derived from alcohol in excess of your energy requirement is simply stored as body fat.

Always remember that high alcohol consumption can damage the liver.

ACTIVITY

Look at your own diet: how much carbohydrate, protein or fat do you eat? How could you improve your diet without making major changes?

KEY TERMS

You need to know what these words mean. Go back through the chapter or check the glossary to find out.	Energy Nutrition Carbohydrate Fat	Protein Alcohol Vitamins Minerals	Trace elements Dietary fibre Water

10 Setting up in business

After working through this chapter you will be able to:

➤ demonstrate an understanding of the options available to you
➤ devise a plan of action
➤ put together a feasibility study/business plan
➤ market yourself.

Once you have qualified as a sports therapist the real work starts – as well as continuing to update your studies, you need to give some thought to just what you are going to do with your new skills.

Sports therapy, although hugely popular, is still relatively new – and for that reason there is as yet no traditional path for graduates to follow. Many finish their courses not knowing what to do or even how to go about using their talents. In this chapter we will look at two options:

1 Employment
2 Self-employment.

Employment

Current opportunities are few, although thankfully the situation is improving. The idea of the sports therapist working alongside the physiotherapist is a romantic idea and not terribly realistic. The sports therapist in employment needs to consider a number of areas, where their skills and expertise might prove useful.

Leisure centres

Council-run leisure centres have a duty to provide the very best facilities to their customers. As a sports therapist you should be capable not only of treating injuries but also of instructing people in a whole range of health and fitness areas. The combination of the traditional 'leisure skills' and extra skills can only enhance your value and worth in this community. You can find information about your local leisure centre from the council or information centre.

Health and fitness clubs

This boom industry is constantly looking for new ideas, each centre being desperate to offer something different that their competitors can't. As a sports therapist you might just be the person they need to enable them to offer a complete range of complementary services. You must push the value of your knowledge – remember you are very capable of offering the following services:

- fitness assessment
- fitness programming
- advice on how to prevent injury
- treatment of injury
- prescription of remedial exercise
- assessment of diet
- knowledge of first aid
- basic business management.

Look in the local telephone directory for contacts.

Cruise lines

Many international companies now see the value in taking a multi-talented sports therapist with them. This is a very specialised market but one well worth looking at. Remember your many different skills. Contact all of the major companies – your local library should have access to a directory giving their addresses.

Working with other therapists

As the news spreads about the good work sports therapists are doing, other therapists who started their own business are beginning to think about employing other people.

<table>
<tr><td>

REMEMBER

No one 'owes' you a job: you really must go out and sell your many talents. It is of no use going to a leisure centre and saying that you are a sports therapist looking for a job – chances are most people won't know exactly what a sports therapist is.

</td></tr>
</table>

Setting up your own business

This is probably the most popular course of action. First, you must be certain that there is a market for your business and that you can offer something that few others are currently offering. Once you are sure of the market you need to consider the following points.

- The size of the business: one room at a health club or a building of your own?
- What equipment will you need?
- How will you market yourself?
- Legal requirements – insurance, industry codes of practice, regional bye-laws relating to your kind of business.
- Will you need help with finance?

What size of business?

You don't need to have plush and expensive premises to run a business. Most sports therapists start by working from home or as a mobile practitioner. Alternatively, you might approach a local health club about renting some space within their building, giving you the opportunity of being self-employed and them the opportunity to advertise your services to their members. Maybe you'll want to invest large amounts of money in your idea and open premises of your own.

Whichever route you choose the basic principles of setting up and running your business are the same.

Equipment you'll need

You will know just what equipment you'll require, and must decide whether to invest in a complete range of the latest and most expensive of pieces of equipment or to use everyday things in order to cut down on costs. Here is a list of 'probable essentials' (this list is meant only as a guide and is by no means intended to be definitive)

- treatment couch (fixed or mobile)
- towels
- couch roll
- cushions
- handwashing supplies
- record cards
- diary
- telephone/answer machine
- car (if you are working as a mobile unit)
- bandaging and strapping
- fitness testing equipment
- rehabilitation equipment.

Your start-up kit really does depend on the type of practice you intend having. Remember, people will use you because of the results you obtain – not because you have the fluffiest towels.

Marketing your business

Expensive newspaper advertising, while often effective, is not the only option. Word of mouth is by far the best form of advertising. Other alternatives include handouts, brochures and posters. Personal contact with sports clubs and athletic associations is also a very good way of promoting your business.

Legal requirements

An area often overlooked when setting up a new business is that of the law and all it entails.

Local bye-laws

Must councils will have some form of legislation about setting up and running businesses providing a 'therapeutic' service to the general public. Your local council offices or local Health and Safety Officer will be able to advise you.

Health and safety requirements

If you are moving into premises you should ask the Health and Safety/Environmental Health Officer for your local council to check your premises and certify them fit for the purpose. These departments have very strict rules and businesses are checked frequently. This is not a bad thing in that obtaining Health and Safety/Environmental Health approval gives your business some official protection.

> **REMEMBER**
>
> *It cannot be emphasised too much that you all should have insurance, whether you are mobile or in exclusive private practice.*

Insurance

Insurance is *essential* for both therapists and their patients. Your insurance should cover both public liability and personal accidents. You must make sure that the cover is adequate for the risks you (and others) may face in your practice. For example, if you are a microlight pilot, it wouldn't be much use taking out an insurance policy that excludes flying.

Insurance cover is not an area in which it is wise to cut corners. Be sure to give full details of all of the services that you are providing. The insurance cover could be invalidated if you fail to disclose any relevant information.

Some validating bodies offer insurance at very competitive rates. It is, however, worth asking an insurance broker to look at the cost of tailoring a policy for you.

Finance

Obviously, the level of finance required depends on a good many things: size, the equipment you require and your personal financial position.

Borrowing money is an expensive business. By far the best route in the early days is to try to remain completely self-sufficient – start small and build your finances while learning about professional practice. You can apply for a career development loan, which, although it must be repaid, has somewhat less restricting terms and conditions than a commercial loan.

Either way, it is a good idea to put together a feasibility study or business plan. This doesn't need to be an elaborate document – in fact it is best kept simple, giving clear and concise information.

The plan

Your business plan/feasibility study should always start with a list of contents; this enables people to find just what they want, without wading through masses of information. It should cover the following areas:

- summary
- personal history
- the market
- management and organisation
- operational plan
- facilities and equipment
- financial plan
- appendices including a curriculum vitae.

Summary

The summary is a crucial part of any plan. Most readers will make up their minds on whether to continue reading from the impression your summary gives them.

Your summary should provide a clear (and very short) view of the main business and the market and should outline:

- *The business*: Briefly describe a business profile, note your main activities, when you wish to start, who is going to own the business, its place in the market, whether there is any competition and any objectives you might have.

- *The type of services you will offer*: Describe what you'll be doing – sell *all* of your skills. Emphasise any advantages that you think you might have over possible competitors. Remember that any potential investor is after a 'winning product'. If the product is you, they must be convinced of your ability.
- *The market and opportunities*: Who are you targeting this business at? What size is that market?
- *Financial highlights*: give a *short* description of any highlights that you might foresee. Your financial highlight might well be that the company was started without any outside finance. Try to give any potential investor a clear picture of business potential and opportunity.

Personal history

Who are you? What is your background? Why did you decide to study sports therapy? Tell them anything relevant – involvement with sports, playing, coaching: anything that gives a clear picture of your suitability for the job.

The market

Who is this business aimed at? Give facts and figures detailing the population of the area the business covers, numbers participating in sport etc. Your local council or library should be able to give you help and advice when compiling this information. Tell the investor how you intend to sell your business.

Management and organisation

This plays a large part in the key to your success. If you are the only person involved then you *are* the management. You must give a detailed account of your personal responsibilities, your experience in these areas and any qualifications to demonstrate your ability to manage your own business.

If you intend to take a part-time business course, then put it in the plan. Let your potential investors know that you are serious about your business and will update you knowledge and skills as appropriate.

If you intend to employ other people, note what their roles and responsibilities will be.

Operational plan

As a service provider you should include a list of your services and details of any facilities and equipment you will have/use. This plan should give details of any equipment you already have and any equipment you need to buy, including when and the cost.

The financial plan

This should be as simple as possible and should be broken down into three different areas.

1 Set-up costs. This should be a detailed list of *everything* you need to set up in business – from advances on the rent to the cotton wool you'll use.

REMEMBER

Keep your knowledge up to date – ideas change and things quickly become outdated.

153

2 Weekly running costs. This needs to be a detailed chart of the actual expenditure you will be committed to – rent, council tax, insurance, heat and lighting, telephone, advertising, cleaning and maintenance, wages, etc.

3 Projected earnings. This is more difficult – and some people would argue it is a pointless exercise. However, it is something that you do need to consider. Very simply, look at the services you intend to provide and cost them out. Once this is done you need to establish the number of general 'treatments' you can complete in any one day. For example:

45-minute treatment (regardless of what it is)	£15.00
Number of treatment slots in an 8-hour day	×7
Potential daily income	£105.00
Number of days each week you'll be working	×5
Potential weekly earnings	£525.00

You will be very lucky if you work to your full potential from the beginning. As a general guide you should work on 30–65% of this.

At 30% the weekly income would be	£157.50
At 40% the weekly income would be	£210.00
At 50% the weekly income would be	£262.50
At 65% the weekly income would be	£341.25

This gives you an idea of the level of business you need to do to cover your weekly running costs/overheads.

This information together gives you a simple but readable financial plan, something to give potential investors an idea of the potential and for you to look at the feasibility of your plans.

Appendices

You should include a copy of your curriculum vitae and that of anyone else you intend to employ or work with.

Some useful addresses

IIST
46 Aldwick Road
Bognor Regis
West Sussex
PO21 2PN

ITEC
10–11 Heathfield Terrace
Chiswick
London
W4 4JE
Tel: 0181 994 4141

British Association of Sports Medicine (BASM)
Education Office
The Anatomy Building
Medical College of St Bartholomew's Hospital
Charterhouse Square
London
EC1M 6BQ

Glossary

Abduction – Movement of a part away from the body
Adduction – Movement of a part towards the body
Analgesia – Decrease in the sensation of pain without loss of consciousness
Analgesic – A drug that produces analgesia
Anoxia – Lack of oxygen
Anterior – Situated towards the front
Anteversion – Tilting or displacement of a body part forward
Articulation – The process of being united by a joint or joints
Atrophy – Reduction in size of a muscle or region of the body; wasting away
Avulsion – Pulling away
Blood serum – Plasma minus its clotting proteins
Bursa – A small sac filled with synovial fluid that allows muscle or tendon to slide over bone
Chondromalacia – Softening and destruction of the cartilage covering the articular surfaces of bone
Chondrocytes – Cells of mature cartilage
Contralateral – On the opposite side
Crepitus – A grating sound or feeling sometimes found in fractures, tendonitis and joint injuries
Cytoplasm – A substance that surrounds organelles
Dense – Thick and compact
Dislocation – Displacement of one or more bones of a joint totally out of the natural joint position
Distal – Furthest away from the centre or midline of the body
Distensibility – Ability to swell
Dorsiflexion – Bending the foot towards its upper surface
Ecchymosis – Bleeding visible beneath skin, causing blue or purple discoloration
Elliptical – Oval
Endosteum – The membrane that lines the marrow cavity of bones
Endomysium – Invagination of perimysium, separating each individual muscle fibre
Endorphins – The body's natural pain inhibitors
Endothelium – The tissue that lines blood vessels and lymphatic vessels
Epiphyseal – Responsible for the lengthways growth of long bone
Epithelium – Tissue that forms glands or outer part of skin and lines blood vessels
Eversion – Turning outwards
Extension – Straightening out of a flexed joint
Extensibility – Ability to extend
External rotation – Rotation of a body part away from the midline
Fascia – The fibrous tissue between muscles, forming the sheaths around muscles and other structures such as nerves and blood vessels
Fibrinogen – A high-molecular-weight protein in blood plasma

155

Fibrin – An insoluble protein that is essential to blood clotting
Fibrous bonds – Bonds that allow little or no movement
Fibroplasia – Process of wound repair
Fasiculus – A small bundle or cluster, especially of nerve or muscle fibres
Flexion – Bending of a joint
Granulocyte – A type of white blood cell
Haemarthrosis – Blood within a joint
Haematoma – A collection of blood, usually clotted, which forms a mass within the tissues following trauma to the blood vessels
Haemorrhage – Escape of blood from blood vessels through damaged walls
Haematopoeisis – Blood cell production; occurring in red bone marrow
Histamines – Chemicals released when cells are injured; result in vasodilation, increased permeability of blood vessels
Hypertrophy – An increase in size of a body part
Hypothermia – Reduction of body temperature to below normal; slows physiological processes
Hypoxia – Oxygen deficiency
Immunological – Protective function
Inflammation – The reaction of tissues to injury; characterised by heat, swelling, redness and pain.
Internal rotation – Rotation of a body part towards the midline.
Inversion – Turning inwards
Lateral – Away from the midline of the body
Ligament – A band of flexible tough fibrous tissue which connects bone to bone within joints.
Lymphocyte – A type of white blood cell found in lymph nodes, associated with the immune system
Manipulation – Skilled use of hands to move joints and muscles. A treatment technique used to obtain forced passive movement of a joint.
Medial – Towards the midline of the body
Metabolism – The sum of all the biochemical reactions that occur within a cell
Metabolic rate – The speed at which metabolism occurs
Microtrauma – Minor, insignificant injury which, if occurring repeatedly will give rise to an obvious injury
Monocytes – A type of white blood cell
Motor nerve – A motor neurone together with the muscle fibres it stimulates
Neuromuscular – Pertaining to both nerves and muscles
Obliquely – Slanting or indirect
Oedema – Excessive accumulation of fluid in tissues and joints
Organic – Derived from living organisms
Osteoarthritis – A degenerative disease affecting joints
Osteoblasts – Cells responsible for synthesis, deposition and mineralisation of bone; mature osteoblasts can develop into osteocytes
Osteoclasts – Cells responsible for removal of bone tissue
Osteocytes – The main cells forming the structure of bone, responsible for maintaining bone structure
Pain free – Before the onset of pain
Parathyroid glands – One of four small endocrine glands
Perichondrium – The membrane that covers cartilage
Periosteum – The membrane that covers bone

Perimysium – Invagination of epimysium that divides muscles into bundles

Perivascular – Surrounding blood vessels

Plantar flexion – Bending the foot downwards towards the sole

Podiatrist – A health professional who deals with the study and treatment of feet

Posterior – Situated towards the rear

Pronation – Turning of the palm of the hand downwards; lowering of the arch of the foot

Proprioception – Appreciation of balance, equilibrium and changes in muscle length and joint position; part of the nervous system

Proximal – Near to the body or midline of the body

Psychic – In the mind

Recticular fibres – Extensive network of fibres which are the precursors of the collagen fibres that will make up a fibrous scar

Refractory – Resisting normal treatment measures

Rehabilitation – Restoration of function to damaged areas of the body

Sarcomere – A contractile unit of striated muscle fibre

Sarcolemma – The cell membrane of a muscle fibre

Sarcoplasm – The cytoplasm of a muscle fibre

Sprain – An injury to a ligament

Strain – An injury involving muscle, tendon or the musculotendinous unit

Striated – In parallel lines

Subluxation – Incomplete or partial dislocation of a joint

Supination – Turning of the palm of the hand upwards; raising of the arch of the foot

Synovium – Membrane lining the joint capsule, bursa and tendon sheaths; produces the synovial fluid

Taut – Drawn tight

Tendon – A band of fibrous tissue attaching muscle to bone

Tensile strength – Strength at the moment of tension

Trauma – Injury to tissue caused by a mechanical or physical agent

Undulating – Moving up and down like waves

Unilateral – On one side

Valgus – An abnormal turning away from the midline of the body or, as in genu valgum (knocked knees), an abnormal turning inwards

Varus – An abnormal turning inwards towards the midline of the body or, as in genu varum (bow legs), an abnormal turning outwards

Vascular – Pertaining to the blood vessels

Vasoconstriction – Narrowing of blood vessels

Vasodilation – Widening of blood vessels

Villus – Mucosal cells containing connective tissue, blood and lymphatic vessels

Index